Contents

Contributors

Hossam Abdalla (Sam) is an Egyptian, born in Illinois, USA. Mr Abdalla qualified at the University of Baghdad in 1977, obtaining the MRCOG in 1983. He carried out junior gynaecological posts, largely at Stobhill in Glasgow, until 1985, when he began to specialize in his chosen field of infertility, working and training in London. In 1988, he became Co-director of the Lister Hospital Fertility and Endocrine Clinic in central London, and under his direction this has grown into one of the largest fertility centres in the country. Throughout he has been at the forefront of his speciality, pioneering new approaches in both ovulation induction and oocyte donation. One aspect of his research resulted in the birth of Britain's first baby conceived from a donated embryo, which had been frozen, thawed and transferred back to the tubes using the ZIFT technique. Highly skilled at laparoscopic gynaecological techniques, Mr Abdalla is also a consultant gynaecologist working at the Chelsea and Westminster Hospital.

Zelda Abramson has a PhD in sociology and is a women's health counsellor living in Toronto, Canada. Zelda's interest in women's health began in the early 1980s when she worked as a medical social worker on the gynaecological and surgical wards. At that time, she also ran outpatient menopausal information and support groups. Realizing she was limited by her work environment in providing the full information women needed to make informed choices, she decided to leave the hospital and, with a group of other women health professionals, opened a private women's counselling and information centre. Her practice includes psychotherapy, consultations, educational and training programmes, and information and support groups.

Carolyn Allan is a registrar in endocrinology at Monash Medical Centre, Victoria, Australia. She graduated from Monash University in 1990 and completed her basic training in internal medicine at Prince Henry's Hospital and Monash Medical Centre. Following this she spent 18 months working in the Department of Obstetrics and Gynaecology at Northwick Park Hospital, Harrow, Middlesex, initially as a senior house officer and then subsequently as a research fellow in the Menopause Clinical and Research Unit. In 1997, she returned to her training in endocrinology as a registrar at St Bartholomew's Hospital, London, but continued her association with the Menopause Unit as an honorary research fellow. In 1999 she returned to Australia to complete her training in endocrinology.

Janet Brockie is a menopause nurse specialist. She has worked at the John Radcliffe Hospital in Oxford since 1986. Janet writes and speaks widely on the menopause. She is an ex-council member of the British Menopause Society. Janet's main areas of interest in the menopause include alternative therapies, the role of the nurse in supporting menopausal women (both on and off HRT) and targeting women at increased risk of long-term post-menopausal problems. Her interest in alternative therapies for the menopause arose from starting and running the Oxford Menopause Support Group.

Gerard S Conway is a clinical endocrinologist with a special interest in reproductive endocrinology, Consultant Endocrinologist at the Middlesex Hospital in London and Honorary Senior Lecturer, Departments of Medicine and Obstetrics & Gynaecology at University College London. For the past 10 years he has held clinics and directed a research team in the Middlesex Hospital, London. His clinical research interests have included polycystic ovary syndrome and the adult consequences of childhood disorders such as Turner's syndrome, androgen insensitivity and congenital adrenal hyperplasia. Studies in premature ovarian failure focus on molecular genetics and autoimmune mechanisms of ovarian destruction. A particular interest is in the characterization of families in which more than one women has experienced an early menopause. Such families will lead to the identification of genes which cause the inheritance of premature ovarian failure. These genes are likely to provide new insights into the mechanisms of ovarian development.

Jean Coope is a general practitioner in Cheshire who has published original research on the menopause and HRT. She pioneered the prevention of osteoporosis in general practice and was a member of the WHO group on research on the menopause that met in Geneva in 1994. From 1994–97 she was editor of the *Journal of the British Menopause Society* and has written many articles and books, appearing on TV and radio to promote women's health.

Catherine Corp has wide experience in nursing, including three years as Assistant Director of a Licensed Practical Nurse programme, two years as a health worker teacher trainer for a non-governmental voluntary agency in a Cambodian refugee camp and three years working as a paediatric home health and hospice nurse. She started the Premature Ovarian Failure Support Group in the USA in the Spring of 1995. Beginning with a local support group, the group now has both formal and informal groups in eight cities, a quarterly newsletter, a website and a listserv with over 250 subscribers. Catherine is now writing a book on premature ovarian failure.

Myra Hunter is head of Clinical Health Psychology at St Thomas' Hospital (South London and Maudsley NHS Trust) and Senior Lecturer with Guy's, King's and St Thomas' Medical and Dental Schools, London. Specialising in Women's health, she has worked with women in a clinical and research capacity for over 20 years. Her PhD (1988) was a prospective study of women's experience of the menopause. Since then she has published many papers and two books about the menopause including *Counselling in Obstetrics and Gynaecology* (BPS Books, 1994). Her current research interests include fertility, menopause, premenstrual problems, domestic violence and women's experience of gynaecological services.

Andrew K S Kan graduated from the University of Sydney Medical School, Australia, with honours in 1987. He completed his internship at the Royal North Shore in Sydney in 1988 and then served in the Republic of Singapore Navy as a medical officer for two and a half years. He then returned to Sydney to start his training in obstetrics and gynaecology at St George's Hospital. He served as a registrar in obstetrics and gynaecology at Guy's and St Thomas' Hospital in London for a year before joining the Lister Hospital IVF

Unit with Hossam Abdalla and John Studd as a clinical research fellow between 1996 and 1998. During that time he published five papers in peer-review journals and was co-author of many publications and presented his work at the British Fertility Society Meetings during that time. Currently he is the Reproductive Endocrinology and Infertility Fellow at North Shore ART in Sydney, Australia.

Lih-Mei Liao is a consultant clinical psychologist. She coordinates the psychological services for endocrinology and obesity at the University College London Hospitals. Lih-Mei's clinical practice characteristically reflects an integration of social and psychological perspectives. Her research interests and publications are in the psychological aspects of endocrine conditions, including polycystic ovary syndrome, atypical sexual development and menopause, on which she wrote her PhD thesis. She teaches clinical psychologists and other health professionals and consultants to several national self-help organizations. Currently she is seconded on a part-time basis to the charity Weight Concern, where she participates in a Department of Health-funded project aimed to develop multidisciplinary approaches for obesity and related problems.

Agnes Marfo is a freelance writer. She graduated from Birkbeck College, University of London, with a BA Hons in English in 1994. Since then she has undertaken a course in freelance and feature writing and has written articles for publication. She has a strong interest in health journalism and women's issues in general. Agnes is currently working on a series of short stories for women's interest magazines.

Joan Pitkin is a consultant obstetrician and gynaecologist at Northwick Park and St Mark's Hospital, Harrow, where she is Director of the Menopause Clinic and Research Unit. She served for six years on the Council of the Royal College of Obstetricians and Gynaecologists, and for three years on the Editorial Board of the *Diplomate Journal*, the Continuing Medical Education Committee and the CD ROM Editorial Board. She was also Diplomate Officer for the College involved with general practitioner training in this speciality. Joan Pitkin has been re-elected to the Council of the British Menopause Society and is particularly interested in menopause postgraduate education and urogynaecology. She runs a menopause unit with a research interest and lectures widely.

Joan Raphael-Leff is Professor of Psychoanalysis at the Centre for Psychoanalytical Studies at the University of Essex. She is a member of the Independent Group of Psychoanalysis of the British Psychoanalytical Society and in clinical practice has specialized in reproductive issues with some 50 publications in this field, including several books: *Psychological Processes of Childbearing* (Chapman & Hall, 1991); *Pregnancy – the inside story* (Sheldon 1993; Jason Aronson, 1996); *Female Experience – three generations of British women psychoanalysts on work with women* (coedited with Rosine Perelberg) (Routledge, 1997); *and Spilt Milk – psychoanalytic interventions in perinatal depression, breakdown and bereavement* (British Institute of Psychoanalysis, 1999). Professionally, Joan Raphael-Leff is Chair of the International Psychoanalytic Association's Committee on Women and Psychoanalysis; is on the steering committee of the Royal Society of Medicine for Prevention of Puerperal Illness; is a founding member of the UK branch of the Association of Infant Mental Health; and is external consultant to the Anna Freud Centre under-five's section, to the Parent Infant Centre and to various perinatal projects overseas.

Dani Singer is a counsellor and psychotherapist in private practice, and a menopause counsellor at Northwick Park Hospital, Harrow, Middlesex. She has published a number of articles on premature menopause and acted on a consultative basis for a television programme on that topic. She lectures in psychology and sociology and is the Book Review Editor for the *Journal of Fertility Counselling*.

Foreword

A woman suffering a premature menopause arrives early at one of life's rather less alluring destinations. When the accompanying and inevitable infertility is recognized, it is obvious that she alights at this stop burdened with existential problems that may overwhelm her. What does it mean for her health and her plans to become a mother? What has happened and why has it happened to her? What can be done to help?

This book responds to these questions in a way that, in my experience, is unique. Having assembled a team of experts from strikingly disparate disciplines, the editors have neatly balanced their contributions. The book, and the reader too, benefits from insights from modern medical genetics, clinical and therapeutic medicine, complementary medicine, human anthropology, sociology, psychology and psychoanalysis. A rich mixture indeed but, as a clinician to whom many patients with this problem have been referred over the years, I can vouch for the need for a guide through this often distressing terrain.

Why is this condition so difficult to bear? After all, health professionals deal every day with patients with illnesses that are more incapacitating, that may be fatal and for which there may be little that even today's medicine can offer. I think at least one of the answers may lie in what, for many women with a premature menopause, must be an assault on their existential assumptions for the present and for the remainder of their lives. And in these days of high personal expectations, in which women have progressively obtained control over so many intimate aspects of their lives, the feeling of being cheated can be dreadful.

This book provides us with a framework of meaning with which to help our patients (who incidentally reappear in some chapters as clients, so no one need fear that an exclusively medical model has been applied). Readers have before them in Chapter 2, a clearly written account of the causes of premature ovarian failure (predominantly genetic so far as they are known at present), and in Chapters 7 and 8, accounts of the clinical assessment and problems of certain specific medical conditions and the optimum schedules of hormone replacement treatment. In Chapter 9 there is an authoritative account of fertility treatments that are possible for the patient with premature ovarian failure. The authors do not dodge very difficult issues, such as the way modern technology, breathtaking as it is in its scope and efficacy, deconstructs traditional notions of motherhood. In this chapter, there is also an illuminating discussion of the ethics of these procedures. Here one also finds the authors' thoughts on what one might tell a child born as result of donated eggs or embryos. Two major issues are considered: the first is parental secrecy and the second donor anonymity. Generally speaking, secrecy in medicine has been abandoned, at least consciously, and I think few mourn its passing. There is little to commend in living a lie and one imagines progressive access to clinical records will make it an increasingly hazardous strategy. I think that maintaining the anomymity of gamete donors is, however, another form of secrecy, one that is presently sanctioned by law and, in the UK at least, promulgated by many infertility specialists. I am uncomfortable with it: knowledge of one's provenance seems to me a right and I have not yet heard arguments sufficiently persuasive to abrogate it. Clearly any change to the regulation of information available to people born as a result of gamete donation could only operate prospectively; guarantees of anonymity given to donors in the past have, of course, to be honoured.

Naturally women differ in their reaction to the news that they have suffered a premature menopause. In Chapter 5 Joan Raphael-Leff describes her notion of generative identity, that is, one's construction of oneself as a potential progenitor. How an individual responds to her loss of fertility will reflect, in part at least, difficulties experienced during the time this identity was acquired. In people whose generative identity is entirely embedded in reproduction, one can readily see how having a child becomes the only route to fulfilment. I can remember as if it were yesterday a young woman about to go to Cambridge University bursting into tears when I told her the diagnosis. What a waste, she sobbed, what a waste. For such a person, despair over infertility can engulf all aspects of creativity.

The psychological and social dimensions of menopause (Chapter 3), the experience of it (Chapter 4) and the diversity of its ethnic content (Chapter 6) are all explored in a remarkable series of chapters. I have mentioned the detail with which medical treatments are described. Not neglected is the approach through complementary medicine (Chapter 10). Here I feel obliged to mention, as does the author of this chapter, that this is a branch of healthcare where the contemporary emphasis on clinical evidence, that is to say, on the rigourous evaluation of treatments in randomized controlled trials, has yet to make much of an appearance. But it is something our patients frequently ask about and so finds a place in this book. Experience of self-help and support groups are described in Chapter 11. The book contains a useful list of contacts, both real and web-based.

Myra Hunter and Dani Singer conclude this book with an account of a biopsychosocial model, an approach which emphasizes the diversity of influences that determines one's response to health problems. Based on this model, they offer some practical advice to healthcare professionals, which will I think enrich our contact with our patients. They identify a number of problems women with premature menopause commonly experience in communicating with their physicians. It is humbling to learn how frequently patients experience their doctors as underestimating the loss they have suffered. But I do often wonder the extent to which the protection afforded by denial in the end limits comprehensive patient–doctor communication.

In many medical situations the professional has but a restricted repertoire of responses. *Premature Menopause: a multidisciplinary approach* leads one away from this limitation and for the first time offers the reader a full and integrated account of this distressing and common condition.

Howard Jacobs
Emeritus Professor of Reproductive Endocrinology
Royal Free and University College School of Medicine
University of London

Preface

Anatomy is destiny
(Freud 1924)

Our bodies set us limits – is there any use in protesting or should we accept the 'natural' order of things? Menstruation and menopause are unique-to-women experiences that all women share. Located at the intersection of women's inner and outer worlds, these two biological events define women as sexual beings, both to themselves and others. Overlaid by social constructions and 'normal' expectations, they strike at the heart of female identity. As pre-pubescent children, girls tend to be accorded a greater freedom than after they begin menstruation, the signal for their being harnessed for the social good and their reproductive function. At menopause, their role is again redefined (primarily as on the way down), their social 'function' more nebulous. Despite recent more emancipatory discourses, these societal prescriptions tend to become lodged deep within every woman's psyche.

In many ways the topic of menopause has come out of the closet, but much remains hidden, unacknowledged and unsaid. Most of the discussion occurs at either the level of physiological symptomatology or on a political, social or cultural level. Psychological implications have been touched on but remain disputed. Numerous studies claim that there is no psychological 'syndrome' unique to the menopause. Nevertheless, there remain popular misconceptions of what it is to be menopausal – if it is not a disease but a natural transition, maybe one is somehow betraying other women if it proves to be problematic.

Each woman, when confronting her own menopause, seems to enter a kind of 'no-woman's' land. Perhaps this is because menopause occupies a place in between contemporary discourses of what being a woman is all about. It has been expressed as: 'am I mad?' or 'is it really "real"?', or something 'hormonal' that can be 'fixed' – 'I know it's supposed to be a natural transition and not a disease, but how come I feel so awful and alone?'

To the extent that this is true for women in general going through 'the change', it is even more so for women with a premature or early menopause. This book hopes to throw some light on these questions in relation to young women who find themselves categorized as menopausal before their 'due' date. Although this book is aimed largely at health professionals, and hence is somewhat academic in its approach, we have also tried to make it readable for women with premature menopause who take an active interest in their condition.

Introduction

I am 38 years old and, having undergone years of unsuccessful fertility treatment, have now been told that I am beginning to go into an early menopause.

As you can imagine, the diagnosis is quite a surprise: I had not expected it to happen yet, and at this age it seems hard to believe.

Early menopause is not something that is easy to talk about and I feel in a bit of a vacuum.

(Karen, excerpt from a letter)

Often, where there are no firm logical connections between material events, we tend to actively construct them, endeavouring to show that what is happening is not random. Deviations from the expected script, especially in relation to the life cycle, present particular challenges.

The worst thing is not knowing why. There's always a secret hope that miraculously it will all start working again.

(Deidre, 26 years)

Until September 1999, with headlines like 'The Menopause is Reversed' (Highland, 1999) followed by a three-page spread, including virtually the entire front page (see also the *Daily Mail*, 1999), an early or premature menopause was still a barely recognized subject. By the late 1990s it had begun to be cited in the psychological literature and in the 1998 *Pennel Report on Women's Health*. News of its existence had gradually started to appear in the media. In Britain, the topic of premature menopause made its television debut in the summer of 1996, presented as part of Channel 4's *Health Alert* series. Entitled 'My Teenage Menopause', it came complete with an accompanying information leaflet. That same year, premature menopause also made a brief appearance on London Weekend Television's *Staying Alive* series. Episode 3, which was billed as 'Cassie receives some shocking news which prompts a violent reaction', showed the character learning that her 'problem' is not cancer but the menopause. 'But I'm only 38', she breathes, and is seen to cry with relief after her doctor tries to comfort her with, 'It's natural, normal...just...a bit early'. Elsewhere screaming headlines such as: 'I had my menopause at nineteen', 'I failed as a woman', 'I'll never have my own children' and 'Finding ways to beat nature's clock', appear with increasing regularity in women's magazines or feature sections of the daily newspapers. Similarly, in the USA, June, the wife of Dr Rex Morgan MD in an ongoing comic strip, is told by her mentor in Nurse Practitioner school, 'June, I started menopause early – in my late thirties' (19 November 1996).

A search on the Internet revealed a busy network of women communicating with each other and seeking information and support. For example:

> I was diagnosed when I was 21 ... I asked her (the doctor) if I could be going through the menopause and she laughed and said no way. I feel like a defective piece of merchandise. I have been told my chance of having another child ... are one in a million...
>
> (Paula, 12 November 1997)

> I can't have a child and you feel so alone
>
> (Lisa, 11 February 1998)

> I walked home in tears ... choice has been taken away ... I had suspected ... that I was menopausal but everyone just wrote me off as being a hypochondriac
>
> (Eli, 19 February 1998)

To date, comparatively little has been written about premature menopause, for women or health professionals. With two notable and recent exceptions (Abernethy 1997b; Hawkridge 1999), only occasionally are there references in the literature to the fact that it exists. Such paucity of accessible information leaves young menopausal women out in the emotional cold and health professionals unfamiliar with its impact.

Physiologically, a premature menopause involves major hormonal changes, which, by themselves, may be difficult to deal with, but they tend to be compounded by pervasive negative sociocultural attitudes towards menopause. Together, these can create distress and concerns that may feel overwhelming, as reflected in women's own accounts (see Chapters 4, 5 and 6).

Despite a burgeoning literature (both professional and popular) on mid-life menopause since the mid-1970s, premature menopause scarcely received a mention. Until recently its existence was acknowledged but the implications remained largely unexplored. In this book we aim to bring together for the first time in a single volume the latest medical, psychological and sociocultural perspectives on premature menopause, a condition that affects some quarter of a million women in Britain today. In this book, a biopsychosocial model is adopted, which aims to give equal emphasis to the influence of biological, psychological and sociocultural factors. It is our view that in order to help women deal with a premature menopause, consideration needs to be given to each of these areas.

The book is divided into three broad sections: the dilemmas of a premature menopause and concomitant bodily changes; how premature menopause is experienced; and treatment approaches. In Part 1, the contemporary dilemmas of a premature menopause are discussed in the context of historical, medical, philosophical and psychoanalytic thinking relating to women. Since many of the fears and myths relating to 'mid-life' menopause seem to exacerbate the impact of a premature menopause, a chapter describing the social meanings of menopause is included together with evidence from recent research which challenges many 'menopausal' myths. In general, women are keen to know as much as possible about the current medical findings relating to their health, including causes and changes affecting their bodies in the short and long term. These issues are addressed in Chapter 2 by Gerard Conway, who goes on to outline current views on etiology, diagnosis, the health implications and prognosis of a premature menopause.

Part 2 begins with women's personal accounts. The emotional upheaval commonly experienced, from the first shock of hearing the diagnosis to medium- and longer-term considerations, is described. Based on an interview study, these accounts are organized thematically to highlight both similarities and variability in the women's descriptions. The psychological impact of a premature menopause is explored further in Chapter 5 by Joan Raphael-Leff. The experience of a premature menopause is highly variable, differing according to social and cultural context. Accordingly, a discussion of the impact of premature menopause within diverse ethnic groups in Britain is discussed by Agnes Marfo in Chapter 6.

The concerns raised and needs expressed by women in Part 2 are considered in Part 3, which focuses on treatment in its broadest sense. It begins with Jean Coope's discussion in Chapter 7 of the management of premature menopause in general practice, usually the first port of call for any woman who notices menstrual changes, fertility problems or vasomotor symptoms, such as hot flushes. This is followed by a consideration of assessment and management of a premature menopause in a gynaecological setting by Joan Pitkin and Carolyn Allen (Chapter 8). Specifically, hormonal treatments with their attendant benefits and concerns in relation to breast screening, bone scans for osteoporosis and cardiovascular disease are addressed. Fertility is an issue for many women with premature menopause; for others, particularly those with children, it may be less relevant. Fertility choices – focusing on the latest developments in egg donation but also including other options such as adoption – are described by Sam Abdalla and Andrew Kan in Chapter 9. Many women today choose alternative treatment approaches, for example complementary medicine. These are described and evaluated by Janet Brockie, a specialist nurse (Chapter 10).

The psychological needs of women can be partially met by provision of clear information and emotional support, and by self-help and counselling groups. Group support can provide a useful forum for sharing information and advice, and can support women by reducing feelings of isolation and offering an opportunity to refocus experience outwards. The sharing that occurs in groups may enable women to challenge unhelpful stereotypes and so develop a sense of control over the situation. This aspect is discussed by writers from England, North America and Canada, who outline ways of starting up and running groups that may encourage readers to do the same.

Finally, we attempt to draw together the themes developed throughout the book. Doctor–patient communication, provision of information and counselling, and the role of supportive services are considered. A biopsychosocial approach is described, emphasizing communication skills and the need for both physical and emotional healthcare.

We hope this book will be useful to health professionals, working at all levels, who are potentially well-placed to raise awareness of premature menopause and mitigate negative attitudes towards it, to provide up-to-date information and offer appropriate help. The challenge for practitioners lies in finding ways of providing broad-ranging holistic services for women with a premature menopause without reinforcing negative feelings of difference, isolation or abnormality.

References

Abernetty (1997b)

Daily Mail (1999) September 23rd p1.

Hawkridge C (1999) The Menopause, HRT and You: an up-to-date and practical guide for women of all ages. Harmondsworth: Penguin.

Highfield R (1999) The Daily Telegraph September 23rd pp1–3.

Part 1
Biological, psychological and social dilemmas

Chapter 1
The dilemmas

DANI SINGER AND MYRA HUNTER

Definitions and historical perspective

> I wish I could write out my sensations at this moment. They are so peculiar and so unpleasant. Partly T(ime) of L(ife) I wonder? A physical feeling as if I were drumming slightly in the veins: very cold, impotent and terrified. As if I were exposed on a high ledge in full light. Very lonely...very useless. No atmosphere around me. No words. Very apprehensive...And I know that I must go on doing this dance on hot bricks till I die.
>
> (Woolf 1937)

When events upset the expected sequences and rhythms of life, by happening at the 'wrong' time, they tend to be harder to bear. In the fast-paced, high-tech, Western world, people tend to live time as a schedule into which they must squeeze their lives. That schedule tends to be prescriptive: things must be done or happen at the right time and in the right place. For women undergoing a premature menopause, nature's timetable appears to have simultaneously halted and inexplicably speeded up: hot flushes, uncertainties and fears, sometimes accompanied by constant fatigue – symptoms commonly associated with menopause – are unexpectedly experienced early, that is, prior to mid-life.

The menopause, commonly dated from the last menstrual period, is generally considered premature when it occurs in women aged 40 or under. There have been variations in the medical literature, ranging from onset prior to 35 years (Bjoro 1966; Jones & Reuhsen 1967) or after the age of 43 (Luisetto et al. 1995). However, most health professionals and researchers use 40 as the marker of a premature menopause (Aubard et al. 1997; Conway 1997; Sung et al. 1997). Premature menopause has been reported in girls as young as 13 (Huerta et al. 1995; Schiffman et al. 1997).

Two thousand years ago, menopause at 40 was generally accepted as 'normal' (Amundson & Diers 1970).

> The menstrual discharge ceases in most women about their fortieth year; but with those in whom it goes on longer it lasts even to the fiftieth year, and women of that age have been known to bear children.
>
> (Aristotle ca 350 BC)

It was not until medieval times that authors cited 50 as the average age of menopause (Amundson & Diers 1973), a change often attributed to increased life expectancy (Hall & Jacobs 1991).

Premature menopause in its broadest sense generally occurs either when the cessation of ovarian function leads to the development of secondary amenorrhoea (where menstruation ceases) or when there is no onset of menstruation (primary amenorrhoea). That is, it is thought to have a biological base, based on follicle depletion (Gosden & Faddy 1998). Premature menopause is also known as hypergonadotrophic amenorrhoea, occult ovarian failure or premature ovarian failure (POF). Occult ovarian failure is usually thought of as an early stage of POF (Cameron et al. 1988). Sometimes a distinction is made between POF and resistant ovary syndrome (ROS). In the latter the ovaries still contain follicles but are inactive (Olivar 1996), whereas in POF the follicles are depleted (see Chapter 2 for more details.)

A medical distinction is made between a naturally occurring menopause and an iatrogenic one – that is, one induced through medical intervention whether surgically, chemically or by radiation. However, the psychological implications – of emotional confusion, physical discomfort and often grief in response to infertility – are probably not affected by these distinctions.

One of the earliest medical cases, reported by Kisch in 1920, was of a young Hungarian woman, aged 17 (Hamblen 1939). At approximately the same time, one of the first mentions of a woman having a premature menopause occurs in the psychoanalytic writings of Helen Deutsch. A classic psychoanalyst who viewed menopause as 'woman's last traumatic experience as a sexual being', Deutsch described a 35-year-old woman who had menopaused who:

had the conscious feeling that this was connected with the approaching maturity of her son...her...fear of incest had caused her to take refuge in an early menopause.

(Deutsch 1925)

By 1950, Arias had reported on 20 women whom he characterized as having an early menopause, although this diagnosis was not fully confirmed. Other 'sightings' in the medical literature followed (Perloff & Schneeberg 1957; Zarate et al. 1970; Starup & Sele 1973), all of which, while recognizing the existence of a premature menopause, simultaneously emphasized its rarity.

The incidence of premature menopause remains relatively rare, but probably 'commoner than generally appreciated' (Ginsburg 1991). Currently estimates range from 1–3% of the female population (Wheeler 1995; Davis 1996) to 10% (Sadler & Syrop 1987). These differences may in part reflect differences in definition. Some distinguish between an early menopause, occurring in women aged 40–45 years, and premature ovarian dysfunction menopause in women under 40 (Crosignani et al. 1998).

The precise nature of premature menopause is hard to pin down. It has been classified as a 'multifactorial syndrome in which genetic, immune and environmental factors may play a role' (Tulandi & Kinch 1981), a heterogeneous condition whose etiology remains elusive in most cases. Although usually thought to be permanent, a few women have been reported to experience spontaneous remissions (Anasti 1998). In two thirds of women, the immune system appears to be implicated, based on an 'abnormal self-recognition' (Hoek et al. 1997). That is, the body's autoimmune system may inadvertently damage the ovary, and possibly other organs such as the thyroid gland, in what has been described as an active form of cell 'suicide' (Billig et al. 1996) or apoptosis – an unfortunate side effect of, for instance, trying to fight infection. Other medical factors cited are: viral infections and abnormal chromosomes (most commonly Turner's syndrome where the X chromosome is missing); or, relatively rarely, fragile-X syndrome, which effectively speeds up the follicle supply a carrier is born with (Kenneson et al. 1997); or other variations on the X chromosome (Barlow 1996). Sometimes genetic and hereditary factors may be involved (Cramer et al. 1995; Cassou et al. 1997; Davis et al. 1998; Vegetti et al. 1998). In addition, environmental factors such as exposure to chemical toxins have also been cited (Silbergeld & Flaws 1999).

Additional etiological theories have suggested that psychological factors may influence early onset. For example, chronic stress, which releases chemicals affecting the pituitary gland, which in turn controls the reproductive system, has been implicated (Vermeulen 1993). Emotional upset, if sufficiently traumatic, can:

> so upset the chemistry of your brain temporarily that the hypothalamus stops working to full capacity.
>
> (Winston 1986)

Individual psychological responses may mediate changes in physiological systems to affect immune function (Laudenslager et al. 1993). Interactions between the immune system and reproduction tend to be complex. For example, if there is build up to high levels of corticosteroids, these could interfere with the release of gonadotrophins. Vinatier et al. (1995) found that immune cells were associated with the regulation of the hypothalamus-pituitary-ovarian axis, either directly or indirectly. However, psychologically related explanations, with regard to premature menopause at least, remain inconclusive.

Cultural experiences

The psychological impact of a premature menopause can be influenced by social and cultural context as well as by material circumstance. An anthropological study carried out in the 1980s found that premature menopause was more common in poor and rural parts of India than in wealthier urban centres (Mahdevan et al. 1982). The difference in prevalence was attributed to material differences in diet, poverty and parity (number of children). In addition, its impact was exacerbated by cultural practices in these rural communities. For example, premature menopause seemingly increased the likelihood of extramarital sexual relations by husbands unhappy at their wives' infertility.

In a later classic ethnographic study of two groups of women, the impact of biocultural factors, such as environment, diet, child-bearing patterns and genetic differences on women's hormonal system, was emphasized. Beyenne (1986) found that among Mayan Indians in Mexico and rural Greek women, generally women experienced the menopause at 35–45 years, with 7% experiencing a premature menopause aged 30 to 35 years. In Mayan culture, early onset was regarded as 'natural for women with numerous children as such women were deemed to have used up their lifetime supply of blood'. Infertility during the reproductive years, however, constituted legitimate grounds for divorce, as children represented security for old age. Mayan women tended to see the menopause as a desirable time of life, free from earlier taboos and restrictions. This contrasted sharply with the experiences of Greek women, for whom menopause signified ageing and decline. Greek women reported physical symptoms similar to their Western counterparts, although these were not associated with disease. The most salient were age and appropriate life stage – to be pregnant when too old was shameful and embarrassing, both to themselves and their family; to be infertile during childbearing years was considered a misfortune. In both cultures, menopause was expected any time after 30, depending on parity and age at onset of menarche. A premature menopause was regarded as problematic if few or no children had been produced. It was expected to engender health problems, increased irritability and feelings of melancholy. The impact of menopause on women's sense of wellbeing appeared to be affected by the social meanings prevalent in the culture, although timing appeared to depend on differences in diet, levels of physical activity and the number of children born.

In the contemporary cultures of Britain and North America, the social and psychological meanings by which women understand their premature menopause are also likely to impact on the subjective experience of it. The main dilemmas faced by women in this context are considered in this chapter.

A natural transition at an unnatural time?

Psychologically, the three 'm's – menstruation, motherhood and menopause – are almost universally considered pivotal life markers for women. The first signifies entry into the realm of womanhood, the second its ultimate fruition and the last an exit from reproductive life. Since a diagnosis of premature menopause is, by definition, something that happens too soon, it is likely to present emotional challenges. These may manifest themselves as fear or confirmation of being abnormal, loss of self-esteem and a sense of existential 'angst' arising from feeling out of control – of one's self, one's body and one's life plans (Mahlstedt et al. 1987; Daniluk 1988; Weiner 1992).

From our earliest childhood we have been learning to master our life, learning to
overcome chaos. Traumatic events mobilise our fear that the chaos will devour
us.

(Leick & Davidsen-Nielsen 1991)

Any entry into a new phase of life challenges self-identity and self-evaluation to some degree, particularly as identity is not just 'for oneself', but also 'for others' (Goffman 1959; Gilbert 1992). Various studies have shown how adolescents who see themselves as physically different tend to have low self-esteem (Rosenberg 1979), and that females significantly more than male counterparts are dysmorphic, that is, express dissatisfaction with their body shape and weight (Fallon & Rozin 1985; Tiggemann & Pennington 1990) – a phenomenon highlighted in the mass media (Orbach 1998a).

Most people, and young women in particular, tend to measure themselves by comparison to others, especially their peers. Young girls tend to learn disgust and shame towards their bodies early on, often from the time of their first period (menarche). Knowing she is 'on time', 'normal', just like her friends, is comforting, especially at a time when so much is shifting and changing both internally (physiologically and psychologically) and socially. On-schedule young women feel better about their bodies than early developers, who tend to have a negative self-image (Tobin-Richards et al. 1983; Peterson & Crocket 1985). This is significant, since attitudes to menopause are often foreshadowed by feelings about menstruation, perhaps particularly in the case of a premature menopause where the gap between the two is unusually narrow:

My first period, at the age of 12, was an acute embarrassment to me. I remember
my mother going into the next room, and telling my father about it. I wished...
the ground would open up around me. Little did I know that...this self-con-
sciousness would revisit me.... For what I hadn't realized was that this would be
one of the only two real periods in my whole life. The second came a couple of
months later and then there were no more ... my ovaries had packed up...now
shrivelled and of no particular use to me.

(Susan, aged 32, 1997).

Menstruation remains most commonly viewed either with 'antipathy' (48%) or as a necessary evil (27%). Only to a lesser extent (25%) is it seen as non-problematic (Scambler'& Scambler 1993), perhaps not surprising in a context where media representations of menstruation are rarely emancipatory:

> the monthly trauma of menstruation ... in many cases can lead to wildly irrational behaviour.
>
> (*The Mail on Sunday* 4 April 1993)

The earlier the 'change', the more distressing the experience is likely to be. It may also lead to a sense of confusion and injustice in cases where daughters have their menopause either at the same time or before their mother experiences her own. The problem presented by deviation from age norms was underlined in one of the few psychological studies specifically relating to a premature menopause. This suggested that the distress at being out of kilter with one's peers is the single most significant factor, over and above any physiological or social losses usually associated with mid-life menopause, and that this held:

> across race, marital status, education and income and regardless of number of children.
>
> (Lennon 1982)

Women's reproductive time, unlike that of men, is limited. Grounded in a monthly reality of menstruation (or in the case of a premature menopause, its absence), women are perhaps uniquely conscious of living on the knife edge of time – in this sense they can be seen as 'the living sacrifice of time' (Bollas 1995). The female biological clock, in the form of the pituitary gland, has been preset – at least until the advent of methods of assisted reproduction:

> Whereas a man owns the 'freehold' of his reproductive organs a woman has them only on a 'leasehold'.
>
> (Welldon 1988)

Existentially thrown into a race against time, women have had to deal with decisions and issues concerning their intentions and desires regarding parenthood much sooner than their male counterparts. A woman with a premature menopause may believe she has lost the race almost before entering it and simultaneously dropped out of the human race because she cannot reproduce 'naturally' (Woollett 1995).

One of the central psychological dilemmas of a premature menopause is that it is hard to think of it as a natural transition in quite the same way as 'on-time' menopause. All psychosocial transitions challenge self-evaluations, which can be positive or negative, shaped largely by the social context in which they occur. Identified as part of a natural process of self-renewal, such transitions may involve spending time shedding aspects of who one was while not yet having arrived at who one will become (Bridges 1980). Usually, awareness of a premature menopause comes unexpectedly and, because it is not at the 'normal' time, this can influence how a woman feels about herself, triggering self-perceptions of inadequacy and incapacity. In Western cultures particularly, a premature menopause is likely to be viewed as an unwelcome transition with none of the sense of a rite of passage increasingly accorded to mid-life menopause. Complicated by the fact that it happens 'too soon', premature menopause confronts a woman with a number of potential losses, both material and psychological. There may be reminders of more prosaic losses, such as being asked to lend tampons, leading some women to feel they need to carry these to avoid embarrassing explanations. Sometimes women feel watched when playing with friends' children, as if they might over-react. And more generally, children playing in the street or a friend's innocent bemoaning of her monthly periods may hold a very different meaning for a woman with premature menopause.

Another aspect of the emotional roller coaster of premature menopause may lie in the virtually universal tendency to operate on the assumption that there are understandable reasons underlying life events. The apparent randomness of a premature menopause may make it difficult to come to terms with one's new biological status because it throws into question so much of what is taken for granted in what it means to be a woman:

> Suddenly a young healthy adult has a medical label – a devastating stigma – thrust upon them. The one 'at fault' feels neutered, unattractive – a 'freak of nature'.
>
> (Mostyn 1992)

Simons (1995) suggested that it may be psychologically preferable to blame oneself for past 'mistakes', real or imagined. The rationale being that this at least implies some kind of action may be possible in the form of atonement that may lead to a resumption of control over the situation – and this is preferable to viewing oneself as a helpless, if innocent, victim. Whether or not this is the case, implied loss of social status can arouse shameful feelings of being perceived as lesser – by both self and others. These feelings may be activated by the broken dream of having (any or more) children and arise from concerns about loss of physiological and emotional control. When they occur they can have a profound affect on a woman's sense of identity.

This is particularly so in the context of the 'post-modern' industrialized West, where connectedness and individuation appear to have become differentially split down gender lines. Broadly, men have been viewed as the ones who 'do' separateness, while women epitomise connectedness. It has been suggested that this variability is the result of different value systems (Gilligan 1982); or because recognition of separation and difference is particularly problematic for women (Sayers 1988); or because women's boundaries are so permeable they tend to end up as mirror images of their mothers (Eichenbaum & Orbach 1983); or because women experience profound taboos against the recognition of their own needs, desires and dependency (Orbach & Eichenbaum 1995). The potential loss of family connectedness can be particularly hard for women whose core identity centres around being able to produce children.

Such lack of cohesiveness and continuity in the experience of self constitutes one of the greatest and most profound sources of anxiety. The psychosocial factors inherent in life changes, particularly those involving close relationships or impinging on social status, have a significant impact on self-esteem (Andrews & Brown 1995) and are likely to play a significant part in a premature menopause.

Fertility and motherhood

A premature menopause causes bodily changes, the symbolic significance of which impacts on areas central to definitions of the ideal woman and encompasses all aspects of sexuality. Young women have a tendency to associate menopause with old age and the end of sexual life, perceptions that potentially impinge on intimate relationships (Bertrand-Servais et al. 1993). This may be reflected in the dilemma regarding their own acceptability expressed by a number of women with a premature menopause, often expressed in relation to disclosure: who to tell and when.

Closely related to sexuality is fertility. Almost universally, religious, cultural and social values set a high premium on fertility. Words such as 'barren', 'sterile' and 'infertile' hold stigmatizing connotations of being unproductive and useless, inviting a sense of failure and worthlessness that is common in almost all cultures.

> To come to terms with disappointment and accepting childlessness are particu-
> larly difficult with the social expectations of our society.
>
> (BMA 1996)

> The last time I failed, I felt quite suicidal. My brother's seven years older. He's
> had children by several relationships. I find this very hard. Even one of his chil-
> dren has had a child – it's so easy, so unthinking for them.
>
> (Deidre, 26)

Many women experience premature menopause before having children, others before they have completed their families. In either situation, the inability to procreate in the traditional manner brings
emotional challenges, which can engender feelings of inadequacy
and isolation. Infertility has been associated with high levels of
distress in otherwise psychologically robust women (Downey &
McKinney 1992) and possibly depression (Domar et al. 1992), a
finding that appeared to be corroborated in some women with
premature menopause (Wood 1996).

The dilemmas surrounding fertility decisions are many and
varied:

> Don't do it too early; don't leave it too late. Don't do it before you're properly
> settled. Don't have an unwanted child; don't have an abortion. Don't be a single
> parent; don't miss out on the joys of childbirth. Don't do it alone; don't let
> strangers rear your children. Don't have a child for selfish reasons; don't be self-
> ish and not have a child. Don't end up in barren solitude; don't expect fertility
> treatment to work.
>
> (Bennett 1996)

Having a child or not is not a private affair but a matter of social
concern. There continues to be considerable pressure to have children (Forrest & Gilbert 1992), while, at the same time, the stigma of
going against nature may be associated with assisted reproduction,
often accompanied by prescriptive notions of what constitutes the
'right' age for motherhood. Literature on the issues faced by people
confronting infertility is rapidly expanding (e.g. Leiblum 1997;
Cooper-Hilbert 1998; Deveraux & Hammerman 1998).

For a woman confronted with a premature menopause, feelings
of having her future stolen from her may arise. 'Natural' (if not
actual) fecundity is now past; biological limitedness has suddenly
become a far more immediate reality than for mid-life counterparts.

If she has not begun to contemplate having children, the experience has the potential to leave her feeling cheated, angry and possibly traumatized. An unmarried or very young woman without a regular partner, may face particular difficulties in establishing intimate relationships, anxious about if, when and how to inform a partner of her condition.

An ancient German proverb held that women should confine themselves to 'Kinder, Kueche und Kirche' (children, kitchen and church). Today, motherhood is still considered a natural and inevitable function of a woman and constitutes a socially sanctioned source of self-esteem and identity. Relatively few women, although perhaps an increasing number, particularly among the highly qualified, choose not to become parents primarily because they have high expectations about the demands of being a parent and are reluctant to take the risk (McAllister & Clarke 1998). Nevertheless, an idealized motherhood is the sometimes oppressive icon all women remain defined against, and in relation to which they tend to define themselves. It continues to be identified as central to what it means to be a woman (Forna 1998).

The cultural allure of motherhood can make coming to terms with childlessness particularly painful (Pines 1993), at the same time as it effectively downplays the diversity of women's ideas and experiences (Phoenix et al. 1991). While contemporary women are more likely to view motherhood as one of a range of identities rather than as their singular and central concern, motherhood and fecundity remain at the core of what is perceived to be a correct 'performance' of womanhood:

> Becoming woman is something women do rather than something women are. In order to 'do girl' women have to negotiate the scripts of femininity which are currently in play and then negotiate the contradictions and inconsistencies. Women have to find a fit between what they want ... and what they are supposed to be.
>
> (Ussher 1997a)

Having children has multiple meanings, which coexist and amplify each other. Children offer one a place in history and may represent an attempt to ascribe meaning to life. They may be seen as extensions of self; those who will rectify past errors, narcissistic adornments and opportunities to make a difference in the world (Rubin 1993). Confronted with being unable to reproduce easily, a woman's self-concept may be undermined (Johnson 1996), despite feminist urging to the contrary (Schover 1994). Being female remains identified with doing what all women are supposed to do, and if for any reason a woman cannot, she may feel diminished.

At one time adoption was considered a route to becoming a (social and legal) parent. In the UK this has become an increasingly less available option as adoption services consider themselves as providers of good homes for children (not necessarily babies) rather than as child-providing services for adults (Blyth 1995). In addition, adoption is often viewed as a less desirable option now that a baby and at least partial genetic relationships are possible (Daniels 1994). Unable to have both options available to them at the same time, and often having to justify an already vulnerable sense of self to those with the power to grant or withold adoption or infertility treatment, can be particularly upsetting:

> It seems unfair that you can't sign up for IVF and adoption at the same time, given the long waiting periods. And it's unfair to be tested as to whether or not you'll make good parents – natural parents don't have to do it.
>
> (Deirdre 26)

Currently, a woman who wants children or wishes to complete her family is increasingly likely to pursue the avenues opened up by reproductive technologies. (see Chapter 9).

Menopause is a probability diagnosis and does not always mean permanent infertility. There has been extensive debate regarding the rare occasions women with a premature menopause have become pregnant spontaneously (Letterie et al. 1990; Jacobson et al. 1991; Gossain et al. 1993; Chen & Chang 1997), chances that may be improved by the use of hormone replacement therapy (Jamin et al. 1995) or therapies that modulate the immune system, such as high dosages of corticosteroids (Hoek et al. 1997). There are also claims that occasionally a premature menopause is reversible or goes into remission, removing barriers to pregnancy (Eden 1993; Busacca et al. 1996). Some studies have suggested that ovarian activity may occur sporadically as ovarian follicular activity may continue (Nelson et al. 1994) and that for a small number of women for whom this is the case there may be a slim potential that fertility can be stimulated (Mehta et al. 1992).

New advances in modern science and conceptual technology are rapidly stretching physiological boundaries. Tantalizing promises that the menopause, i.e. biological limitations, may soon be 'abolished altogether' have been put forward for some time (Gosden 1996). In 1999 this idea seemed to turn into a real possibility when a 30 year old woman with a premature menopause underwent an ovarian autograft. The young woman had an ovary removed when she was 17 because of a cyst; at 29 she had a second ovary removed to treat what was described in the newspapers as a 'benign medical condition' and – at her request – the tissue was frozen. The ensuing autograft, designed primarily for young women undergoing treatment for cancer, seemed to suggest that in theory some young women might be offered an opportunity to have their own genetic child by storing their ovarian tissue in thin slices in liquid nitrogen, to be grafted back later (Gosden et al. 1999). Potentially this treatment offers hope to those young women who can predict their menopause because it is medically induced. For the majority of women with premature menopause, for whom diagnosis is after the event and whose ovaries no longer contain sufficient eggs, such news may be unhelpful. Nevertheless, this serves to fuel 'hope in the freezer' (Leadbetter 1997) and the possibility of 'reproductive insurance' (Wood et al. 1997). While extensive media coverage plants seeds of hope and raises women's expectations, including those of older women (Maggs-Rapport 1998), at the time of writing the technique remains unproven and ethically controversial, in the UK at least. Increasingly, infertility is seen as a temporary state, more a social construct than a medical condition, as infertility treatments become more commonplace (at least for those who can afford them) and used even when there is no medical need for treatment (Koch 1998).

Rapidly evolving fertility treatments using ovum (egg) donation can considerably boost the figures of pregnancy rates for women with a premature menopause. At the time of writing estimates varied from between 20% and 30% (Morris & Sauer 1993) to 13.9% overall live birth rate per cycle of treatment (Templeton et al. 1996). This variation depends in part on age and duration of infertility as well as embryo quality and the success of the hormonal preparation stage of treatment. Overall, the message is that soon women will be able to choose between accepting loss of fertility or attempting to regain it through assisted conception (primarily ovum [egg] donation for women with a premature menopause and surrogacy for those who have undergone a hysterectomy). However, there is usually a shortage of eggs available for donation, at least in the UK where payment to donors remains prohibited. This has resulted in schemes for 'egg-sharing' between women undergoing IVF and those needing ovum donation, schemes that are not yet widespread (Ahuja et al. 1996, 1997).

While promising a positive outcome for some, assisted conception may not always bring the desired results (Whiteford & Gonzles 1994) or provide a magical solution to the emotional complexities involved. Women report struggling with conflicting information and statistics regarding treatment: the pain of the treatment itself; the enormous disappointment of failure, sometimes seemingly more unendurable when the help of modern reproductive techniques fail, as well as the practical and emotional dilemma of being dependent on a third party. Having a child using ovum donation is often psychologically complex. Unresolved issues around infertility may become subsumed beneath the quest for parenthood at all costs, or they may act as impediments to treatment, sometimes expressed as fears of not looking like or being like their own child:

> I had a chance for egg donation, but the genetic mother did not look at all like me, so there'd be no connection to 'me'. What if I don't like it or don't bond to it? Or if something goes wrong I won't know where that comes from and not only then, even if it's a talent. I still don't know if I want this for me or for my partner.

It was observed over a hundred years ago that women are often willing to submit to intrusive procedures in the hope of relief from infertility (Ashby 1894), and psychologically little seems to have changed (Sandelowski 1991). Technological advances may serve to mitigate the struggle with reproductive limitations but they can also come at a high emotional cost (Goldenberg 1997; Slade et al. 1997, McLean 1999), reinforcing cultural injunctions that equate femininity with reproduction.

Assisted conception is rapidly deconstructing earlier, more fixed notions of motherhood. Today, one woman may become an ovarian supplier, another the uterine or birth mother, and a third the social mother who raises the child, or some combination of the three. At the same time this process can create so-called 'embryonic orphans' with no biological connection to either social parent (Holbrook 1990). The terminology used in the literature of reproductive technology tends to discuss the female body in terms of 'egg harvesting' and 'uterine environments' and this has been criticized for turning women's bodies into virtually living laboratories (Rowland 1987). On the other hand, reproductive techniques can provide a welcome opportunity of overcoming the loss of parenthood caused by a premature menopause, which a proportion of women are keen to pursue.

Medical dilemmas

Women with a premature menopause may feel particularly isolated because their condition is one of the remaining undiscussed topics in women's health. Hidden from the naked eye, a woman may receive little sympathy or recognition either from friends, who do not have similar concerns and may fail to understand how deeply she is affected, or from some of the professionals from whom she seeks medical advice. Further, her condition is likely to be 'medicalized' for much of her life, implicitly positioning her as deficient (of oestrogen which needs replacing) – often at a time when the social expectation is that she should be feeling at her healthiest. Faced with the practical problem of possibly having to pay a lifetime of prescriptions, a young menopausal woman may view both her body and her 'self' as problematic:

> The girl in the ad looks young and attractive. On her taut left buttock is a discrete little patch. Take HRT, it seems to suggest, and you too can be like this. I am also young, but the patch on my bottom is four times the size of the one in the ad. Much less glamorous and with all the eroticism of a sandwich bag.
>
> (Hawkridge 1997)

Repeated visits to a medical practitioner may reinforce an incipient sense of shame, as may invitations to attend menopause clinics. There, a young woman, usually alone among a sea of middle-aged to elderly women, may feel peculiarly out of place and exposed – the more so in a cultural context that encourages young women to identify with (young) men rather than with other, particularly older, women (Sybylla 1997). Thus a woman experiencing a premature menopause may feel she stands out:

> an isolated figure against a bleak relentless ground, the ground of contemptuous and punishing self and others ... thrust outside society ... psychically extinct.
>
> (Pines 1995)

In this context, the language used to describe a young woman's menopausal status is likely to carry profound psychological implications for her self-concept. Much of the medical language used is cast in the negative, in terms of what is missing or lacking, effectively excluding her from the world of natural motherhood and children and offering in its place only a deficiency model of womanhood (Ireland 1993). In a society emphasizing productivity and success, words like ovarian 'failure', 'incompetent' cervix, 'blighted' ovum and 'hostile' mucous can only serve to further undermine an already shaken sense of self-esteem. The medical profession does appear to be taking on board the psychological impact of medical terminology in relation to some conditions, such as pregnancy loss (previously called abortion), and the need for skilful communication (Freeling & Gask 1998; Hutchon & Cooper 1998). Interestingly, a number of women prefer to use the term 'ovarian failure' because it includes women who have had cancer and thereby reduces connotations of something innately faulty.

A further dilemma is that of an 'HRT culture' wherein hormone replacement therapy (HRT) is perceived as being prescribed as a panacea. Resultant media representations have:

> led women to fear their bodies as they reach the change. Tales of hot flushes and night sweats, dried-out vaginas, skins that crumple like a burst balloon, murderous moods and sexual ennui have been written about ad nauseam. The message is that an unbearable and inevitable fate is linked to the process of change.
>
> (Neustatter 1997)

For young women particularly, it is hard to know where they fit in the ongoing debates about the advantages and disadvantages of HRT. The majority of medical practitioners recommend its use as a prophylactic therapy against the increased risk of osteoporotic fractures, cardiovascular diseases, possibly Alzheimer's and indeed against ageing generally (Bagur & Mautalen 1992; Toozs-Hobson & Cardozo 1996; Anasti et al. 1998); others emphasize a more cautious risk-benefit assessment depending on other health factors (Khaw 1998).

For women with premature menopause, hormonal treatment is likely to be a long-term need. The prospect of 20 or more years of HRT is, perhaps understandably, daunting to young women in their twenties and thirties. Recent interest has focused on diet as an alternative to HRT, but on the whole this area of research remains inconclusive (see Chapter 10). It has been suggested that plant-based phytoestrogens, found in soyabean products, grain cereals, seeds, berries and some vegetables, have a protective effect. Japanese women have, for example, been found to have milder menopausal symptoms, possibly because their intake of phytoestrogens in food is higher (Adlercreutz et al. 1998; Lock et al. 1988). Other suggestions for alleviating menopause symptoms, particularly in relation to osteoporosis, are physical exercise, a diet rich in calcium but limited in caffeine, alcohol and protein; and an avoidance of smoking. While diet may assist in the reduction of some of the classic menopause symptoms and possibly in protecting against heart disease (Department of Health 1994), it is not generally considered to adequately address the issue of bone density loss, particularly for women who may need 15 to 30 years' worth of oestrogen supplement. In addition, the HRT picture itself is broadening. There is now a choice of 'natural' or synthetic hormones, tissue-specific selective (o)estrogen receptor modulators (SERMS) and various routes of administration (oral, gels, implants), which can be tailored to individual requirements. The need to allow room for negotiation, consideration of alternatives (e.g. taking phosphates for bone density), monitoring and periodic follow-up consultations with the woman's physician is increasingly recognized (Hillard 1998).

Where premature menopause is surgically induced (as in a bilateral oophorectomy), or arises from chemotherapy or radiation treatments, the physiological experience of menopause may be sharper, more intense and long-lasting, although severity tends to be highly variable. The emotional experience among women who have undergone this operation can be problematic, particularly if the woman was not fully prepared beforehand. Where women experience a premature menopause due to chemical or radiation therapy, emotional reactions tend to be shelved in the face of the need for survival. Only after the initial crisis has passed may issues of living, such as fertility, sexuality and relationships, resurface. Periods that stop abruptly may aggravate feelings of bodily failure and betrayal in women already vulnerable from the shock of having (had) for example, cancer. If accompanied by pain or discomfort in their sexual life, this may interfere with their ability to receive the warmth, affection and sense of acceptability necessary for wellbeing (Cone 1993). This may be particularly poignant in young girls treated for cancer during childhood or adolescence, who need to be made aware of their smaller window of fertility so that they can plan their families accordingly if they so choose (Byrne et al. 1992). In this context, intimate, particularly perhaps heterosexual, relationships can be either difficult to form or painfully disrupted if left unaddressed, and often women are left uneasy, wondering what else in their body might be faulty.

Psychologically, once a diagnosis has been medically established, a woman faces a loss that is simultaneously shadowy and real. The former takes the form of an absence of something that has failed to occur, the result of a disjuncture between biological and social timing; the latter is the material loss of being able to reproduce naturally. Both are mediated by age. For a woman in her early to mid-twenties, whose friends may be having or planning families, seeing images of mothers with their babies – now more than ever present in the fashion magazines – while experiencing possibly distressing hormonal changes, can be immensely painful. For a woman in her early to mid-thirties, who perhaps postponed having children for professional reasons, the same context may hold a different form of psychic pain, such as regret and self-blame at having taken her ability to procreate for granted.

Early ageing

For most people ageing is a gradual, barely perceptible process, making it possible to maintain the illusion that one is the person one thought one was five years ago. In the experience of a premature menopause, a woman's expected trajectory is disrupted. Core beliefs are challenged, jeopardizing her sense of self as continuous. Abruptly ejected from her assumptive world, a woman's construction of who she is may become dislocated (Woodfield & Viney 1982). This view has been supported by Baber et al. (1991), who found that 28% of women with a premature menopause felt they had suddenly aged. Premature menopause may be the first unexpected encounter with mortality, and coming at a time when women are supposed to be feeling at their healthiest; it is perhaps all the more shocking and difficult to absorb for that. Most people go through life denying their own mortality or at least shelving the thought of it – undoubtedly encouraged by a social context in which one is daily bombarded with exhortations on how to stay young, live longer and beat 'your genetic time bomb' for example by dividing the enzyme telomerase to build biochemicallly 'youthful' cells (Radford 1998). If this denial is eaten away in piecemeal fashion, as we all know it must be, it is perhaps easier to accept. But to be confronted with it too soon can be perceived as a mortifying blow, engendering feelings of sadness and possibly depression.

Although a premature menopause is not related to the ageing process per se, menopause at any age is strongly associated with, if not reduced to, ageing (Gulette 1997). Several studies, spanning almost 30 years, have shown that younger women hold a more negative stereotype than older women of what it means to be menopausal (Neugarten et al. 1968; Bowles 1986; Gannon & Eckstrom 1993). This is hardly surprising given media representations that paint a picture of the menopausal woman as irritable, frequently depressed, asexual and besieged by hot flushes (Reitz 1991). The menopausal woman's social undesirability is further reinforced by aggressive marketing of health, fitness, youth and sexuality (Komesaroff et al. 1997). In a sociocultural context wherein mid-life menopause is widely held to be the beginning of the end (Richters 1997), it makes the issues that women with a premature menopause have to confront that much more difficult. While the younger menopausal woman may have the 'advantage' of not actually being old, the social meanings of menopause might lead to her feeling in danger of imminent atrophy. Together, the 'double whammy' of infertility coupled with an expectation of premature ageing, each with their attendant negatively hued sociocultural baggage, form the central dilemmas of a premature menopause.

Individual differences

The personal and social predicaments posed by a premature menopause vary considerably from woman to woman. Women with a premature menopause do not form a single, homogeneous group. As well as significant individual differences mediated by personal history and sociocultural and material circumstances, there may be different impacts depending on the age at which a premature menopause occurs. Developmentally, women with a menopause before age 20 may have barely negotiated young adulthood. Suddenly, they may find themselves face-to-face with issues that usually have more relevance to middle-aged or older women, often without the necessary life experience or adequate social, familial or professional support. Among the over-thirties, many of whom may have children or have made conscious choices to be child-free, the fear of premature ageing and associated health concerns, such as osteoporosis and cardiovascular disease, may seem more immediate than a lack of choice regarding future children. However, for those in this age group who postponed reproductive decisions, a premature menopause can be particularly distressing – a source of regret at lost opportunities.

A growing number of mid-life women experiencing menopause have been viewed as possessing the self-confidence to actively reclaim this time of life as a positive transition for further development rather than experiencing it as a necessary decline (Zachary 1995). Arguably this may be more difficult to achieve for younger women. Any positive sense of renewed freedom or relief from the hassles and expense of periods may be outweighed by feelings of being unacceptably different, abnormal and possibly to blame for their condition. The strength of such feelings is likely to vary according to a woman's personal, social and cultural circumstances as well as her physiological experiences.

In conclusion, the dilemmas of a premature menopause can involve apprehension at deviating from the norm, having a 'medical' problem in the sense of needing ongoing medical treatment, and associated worries about future health and premature ageing. Further aggravated by lack of information and uncertainty, these difficulties intersect with the largely negative social meanings of menopause, which may engender uncomfortable feelings of shame and guilt. Faced with potential losses of natural fertility and self-esteem, personal identity is frequently challenged, particularly at the younger end of the age spectrum. Yet menstruation, motherhood and menopause do not constitute the sum of 'womanhood' and women need not remain confined by social values and practices that attempt to situate them thus. The dilemmas of a premature menopause are a result not only of the personal problems of individual women, but also by the juxtaposition of biological changes, material circumstances and the still predominantly negative social meanings of menopause, infertility and ageing.

Chapter 2
Etiology, diagnosis and prognosis

GERARD S CONWAY

Background

The ovary is unique in the body, being an organ that has a normal duration of function that falls short of modern life expectancy. The menopause occurs when the number of eggs within the ovary reaches a critically low level, the normal cycle of egg maturation ceases and menstruation stops. On average, menopause occurs at the age of 50 (McKinlay et al. 1992a). Around this average age the frequency distribution of menopausal age is normal, with 1% of women continuing to menstruate beyond the age of 60 and 1% whose menopause occurs before 40. Arbitrarily, a menopause before the age of 40 is defined as 'premature'.

The life span of the ovary can be considered in terms of its cellular make up. The ovary is made up of four types of cells. Germ cells mature into eggs. Granulosa cells surround each germ cell to form a primordial follicle, which may mature into an ovulatory follicle if called upon. Theca cells surround each follicle and mature into stroma cells, which fill the centre of the ovary and supporting cells provide fibrous structure to the ovary. As each follicle matures, theca cells produce testosterone, which is converted to oestrogen by the neighbouring granulosa cell. After ovulation the successful follicle turns into a corpus luteum and produces progesterone. Any remaining follicles shrink away as the ovary prepares for the next cycle.

Premature menopause may be caused by any process that reduces the number of eggs within the ovary. In the embryo, eggs first appear as germ cells in the urogenital ridge. These germ cells then migrate to the primitive ovary. Once within the ovary, the germ cells multiply to form 3.5 million potential eggs in each ovary (Baker 1963).

From this time on these eggs are held in suspended animation – meiosis prophase – until required for ovulation, up to 40 years later. This process is, incidentally, very different from sperm production in men, which occurs constantly throughout life. If a woman were to ovulate every month throughout her reproductive life then she would use fewer than 500 eggs – a tiny proportion of the original seven million (0.007%). And if she were to prevent ovulation, say by taking the combined oral contraceptive pill constantly, the age of the menopause would not be affected in any way. The timing of the natural menopause is inherited; daughters tend to follow their mothers and timing is also advanced by environmental factors such as smoking. In most instances, women with a premature menopause depart from this rule as some extraordinary event causes damage to the ovary. The age of menopause has no relationship to the age at which periods start (menarche).

What then does control the number of eggs in the ovaries throughout life? Most eggs are destroyed intentionally by the body through a system of 'programmed cell death' or apoptosis (Hsueh et al. 1994). The body destroys eggs in several stages (Figure 2.1). Before birth, two-thirds of the seven million eggs are destroyed in a very rapid round of apoptosis, presumably effecting a selection of the healthiest eggs. Between infancy and the age of 40, eggs are gradually reduced from approximately one million to 10,000 in each ovary. Around the age of 40 the process of egg destruction is accelerated and few are left by the age of 50. Very little is known about the processes that control these three phases in the life of the ovary but it is clear that eggs are very vulnerable in the state of suspended animation in which they are held until called upon to go forth and ovulate. For example, if there is an abnormality of the X chromosome such as in Turner's syndrome, where one X chromosome is missing, then egg production is normal but the first phase of egg destruction is accelerated, leaving very few eggs available at birth (Singh & Carr 1966). The missing X chromosome appears to destabilize the suspended egg ensuring the early death of the ovary in individuals with Turner's syndrome.

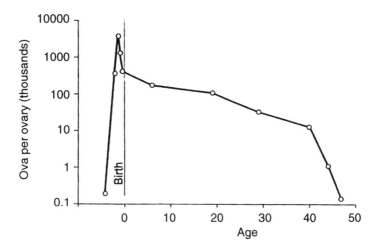

Figure 2.1: Scheme of the number of eggs within each ovary before and after birth, determined by counting germ cells in the ovaries from postmortem specimens.

Terminology

The process of ovary destruction is complex and prolonged. As a result, various components of the process have each acquired different labels, even though distinction between these events is largely artificial.

Ovarian dysgenesis

Ovarian dysgenesis is failure of the ovary to develop. When the ovary is damaged at a very early phase it appears, on examination, to be composed only of streaks of fibrous tissue and in some instances no ovarian remnant can be identified at all. Females fail to enter puberty and never experience spontaneous periods; this is called primary amenorrhoea.

Premature ovarian failure (POF)

In premature ovarian failure the ovaries cease functioning after menstruation has started. The ovary appears to function normally in the progress through puberty and the start of menstruation occurs normally. POF can occur at any age, although it is unusual for teenagers to be affected. Most investigators take a cut-off of 40 years as the definition of premature menopause. This arbitrary age, however, hides the fact that some women with the onset of POF in their thirties have an advanced form of physiological ovarian failure. For this reason, researchers investigating pathological mechanisms might focus on a younger age group.

Resistant ovary syndrome (ROS)

Resistant ovary syndrome is a form of ovarian failure where the ovarian apparatus appears to remain intact (Jones & Moraes-Reuhsen 1969; Dewhurst et al. 1975). Early investigators undertook biopsies of failing ovaries to discover what was going on. In a few instances, microscopic examination revealed normal-looking eggs and ovary structure. They presumed that these eggs were resistant to the reproductive drive of the body – hence resistant ovary syndrome. Disappointingly, the biopsy results helped little in the development of fertility treatment. Most doctors now understand ROS to be a form of partial ovarian failure that usually progresses to the complete menopause in a short time. ROS is also used to refer to the situation when periods continue to occur but blood tests show signs of ovarian failure.

Occult ovarian failure

This describes a lesser form of partial ovarian failure whereby the serum follicle-stimulating hormone (FSH) concentration is raised but menstrual cycles persist (O'Herlihy et al. 1980). Clearly each of these conditions describes one part of a spectrum of ovarian failure but only slightly improves the outlook for fertility.

Hypergonadotrophic amenorrhoea

This collective term encompasses all conditions that present with raised serum FSH concentrations and no periods for six months or more (Rebar 1982). That is, it covers all the terms above except for occult ovarian failure.

Etiology of premature ovarian failure

It is frustrating that the cause of premature menopause is unknown to the majority of women in whom the diagnosis is made. The psychological impact resulting from this diagnosis can be eased by a clear definition of the mechanism involved. Thus even though investigation of the cause rarely leads to altered management, the dividends in terms of coping with the diagnosis are substantial. A list of causes of POF in women attending clinics at the Middlesex Hospital is presented in Table 2.1. In general, the known causes can be categorized into genetic and environmental mechanisms.

Table 2.1: Causes of premature ovarian failure in 352 women attending the Middlesex Hospital

	n	%
Idiopathic (including autoimmune)	204	58
Turner's syndrome	82	23
Chemotherapy	24	7
Familial POF	15	4
Pelvic surgery	8	2
46 XY gonadal dysgenesis	7	2
Galactosaemia	6	2
Pelvic irradiation	6	2

Genetic causes

Any defect of the female sex chromosome – the X chromosome – can cause ovary failure. The most common form is Turner's syndrome. Women with Turner's syndrome have one X chromosome missing giving the chromosomal make-up of 45XO. For comparison, most females are 46XX and most males 46XY. Women with Turner's syndrome are commonly short of stature and do not spontaneously enter puberty. The very early development of the ovary in women with Turner's syndrome appears normal but all germ cells are lost by birth, giving a picture of gonadal dysgenesis.

The paradigm of Turner's syndrome demonstrates that two intact X chromosomes are vital for normal ovarian function (Zinn et al. 1993). From the study of women with partial deletions of the X chromosome, it is clear that at least three loci are critical for ovarian development (Powell et al. 1994). On a short arm of the X chromosome are genes responsible for the stigmata of Turner's syndrome and primary amenorrhoea. Particular interest has focused on Xp22, where there are a series of genes that escape X-inactivation in humans. Among these, the ZFX gene is a prime candidate for an association with premature menopause (Schnieder-Gadicke et al. 1989). ZFX is the homologue of ZFY, which was once a candidate for the testis-determining factor on the Y chromosome. The role of ZFX has recently been clarified by the generation of female ZFX knockout mice with premature ovarian failure (Luoh et al. 1997). Thus, the combination of features of being in a candidate area of the X chromosome, escaping X-inactivation and exhibiting the appropriate knockout phenotype, all make ZFX a prime candidate gene for premature menopause.

The smallest deletions of the X chromosome known to cause premature menopause has identified Xq26-28 as harbouring a gene that may cause POF (Bates & Howard 1990). Centrokmeric to the FRAXA locus (see below) is the SOX3 gene, which has been mapped to Xq26-27.2 and also fulfils several criteria as a candidate for POF. This gene, which also escapes X-inactivation, is the homologue of the SRY gene that determines testicular development in the Y chromosome in males. No mutations of the SOX3 gene have yet been noted. We have recently identified a family that transmits stable deletions of the X chromosome with a break point at Xq26 (Davison et al. 1998). Close analysis of this genetic make-up will allow the identification of new candidate genes in which mutations might lead to premature menopause.

The third area of the X chromosome that is thought to be critical for ovarian development is Xq13-22. Recently, a collection of women with break points located in this region and who present with premature menopause have been studied (Sala et al. 1997). In a region covering 15 megabases, it was estimated that several POF genes must exist. Taken together, these growing data on the X chromosome lead us now to believe that there are not just critical regions on this chromosome but a series of genes any of which might have a mutation and precipitate premature menopause.

In some instances premature menopause appears in several female members of the same family where no cytogenetic defect can be identified (Vegetti et al. 1998). Occasionally, genetic markers can be found that can predict premature menopause in future generations of such families. For this reason a detailed family history is an essential part of the background when considering causes of ovary failure. In most instances the mode of inheritance is not known and much research is being directed at unraveling the genetic pattern in such pedigrees. From the published data on these families, it is clear that familial premature menopause has several modes of inheritance – autosomal dominant, autosomal recessive and X-linked inheritance have all been reported (Coulam et al. 1983; Mattison et al. 1984). Frequently, because of the inherent infertility, the information does not extend far enough back to determine mode of inheritance.

Premature menopause is also present in families with rare inherited conditions such as galactosaemia (a difficulty in utilizing the sugar galactose, which consequently accumulates in the blood), fragile X syndrome and blepharophimosis (a small aperture between the eyelids). In each of these instances, the mechanism of ovarian damage is unknown. In galactosaemia, the vast majority of affected females present with primary amenorrhoea, whereas male fertility appears to remain intact (Kaufman et al. 1994). In blepharophismosis, only one half of families exhibit early menopause, often with the clinical picture of resistant ovaries (Panidis et al. 1994; Fraser et al. 1998).

In families transmitting fragile X syndrome, there is a particularly fascinating relationship with premature menopause. Fragile X syndrome is the most common inherited cause of mental retardation in boys. It is caused by a trinucleotide repeat sequence in the FMR1 gene (Jacobs 1991). Normally fewer than 50 repeats of a CCG sequence occur at this FRAXA site. A full mutation at this site is defined as a repeat number in excess of 200, where the FMR1 gene fails to function and mental retardation ensues. A premutation is an intermediate state, where between 50 and 200 repeats occur. Individuals carrying the premutation were thought until recently to have no phenotype but to be at risk of transmitting fragile X syndrome if the trinucleotide repeats 'expand' into the full mutation range in the next generation. Curiously, premature menopause is associated only with the premutation status – often in the generation before fragile X syndrome appears in these families (Conway et al. 1995, 1998). The clinical presentation is with secondary amenorrhoea between the ages of 11 and 37. Some studies focusing on older age groups have failed to find an association between POF and FRAXA premutations, probably because of the dilution effect of women entering the physiological menopause.

The FSH receptor gene has long been considered the foremost candidate gene for the familial form of premature menopause. That is, if the actions of FSH on the ovary were blocked, then the ovary would fail to develop. In Finland, Ala189Val mutation affecting the extracellular domain of the FSH receptor gene was found to be associated with POF in 22 women from six families presenting with primary amenorrhoea (Aittomaki 1994; Aittomaki et al. 1995, 1996). The ovaries in these women were hypoplastic, with numerous primordial follicles that failed to develop beyond a primitive stage. Interestingly, some of the males homozygous for the FSH receptor-blocking mutation proved to have fairly normal fertility. Extensive studies in other countries have shown that FSH receptor-blocking mutations are a very rare cause of premature menopause.

Environmental causes

In life there are several insults to the ovary that may result in permanent damage and depletion of germ cells. First, the ovary may be affected by medical treatment. Almost any surgery within the pelvis, such as ovarian cyst removal or hysterectomy, might damage the ovary probably by affecting the blood supply or causing inflammation in the area. The risk of ovary failure through pelvic surgery is unknown and thought to be very small indeed for most routine operations. Surgery on more distant organs, such as the appendix, is not reported to damage the ovary, even though related infections might cause infertility through the formation of adhesions between the fallopian tubes and surrounding structures.

As more women survive childhood cancer or leukaemia, we realize that chemotherapy and radiotherapy commonly cause permanent damage to the ovary (Critchly et al. 1992; Clark et al. 1995). It is this group of women who might be offered cryopreservation of ovary tissue before chemotherapy.

Autoimmunity

All glands within the body have a tendency to be damaged by the immune system, the theory being that endocrine organs have epitopes which are closely mimicked by bacteria and viruses. Examples of such autoimmunity are hypothyroidism, adrenal failure (Addison's disease) and type 1 diabetes mellitus. Each of these can occur in conjunction with premature menopause (Weetman 1995). As a general rule the ovary is the last gland to be affected when several conditions are involved. Hypothyroidism in particular occurs more commonly than expected in women with premature menopause, making it likely that in some circumstances the ovary is damaged by antibodies in the same way as the thyroid gland. By analogy, the ovary might also incur autoimmune damage even when no other gland seems to be affected. Unfortunately, current tests are not sufficiently sensitive to determine when this might be the case, but the refinements of these tests is a major drive in current medical research.

Interest in this field arises from the possibility that an autoimmune marker might predict impending ovarian failure. Such a marker might enable prevention of complete menopause if early immune suppression was applied. A very few pilot studies have suggested that treatment with prednisolone might reverse ovarian failure in some women (Blumenfeld et al. 1993; Corenblum et al. 1993). In order to discover who might respond to steroid treatment, several autoimmune antigens have been assessed as predictive markers (Hoek et al. 1997). No such autoimmune test has yet achieved wide application and they remain in the realm of research. One promising marker currently under assessment in our own laboratory is 3 beta-hydroxsteroid dehydrogenase (3βHSD). This steroidogenic enzyme is present in the ovary and in the adrenal gland. Antibodies of 3βHSD are found in approximately 20% of women with premature menopause attending our clinics and the possibility that some of them might respond to steroid treatment is currently under investigation (Arif et al. 1996).

Toxins and viruses

In most women with premature menopause, the mechanism of damage is unknown – there is no family history, the chromosomes are normal and there is no sign of autoimmunity. We might guess that hidden environmental damage has occurred, perhaps in the distant past, leaving no trace by the time periods have stopped. In men, we know that viruses such as mumps can inflame the testicles causing permanent damage and lack of sperm. Similarly it is a popular belief that sperm counts have fallen over recent years because of exposure of the testicles to environmental toxins or drugs. It is likely that the ovaries are affected by viruses or toxins in a way akin to the testes. In particular, viruses are a likely cause of ovarian failure in women for whom no obvious cause is detected. Anecdotal reports of virus infections being quickly followed by ovarian failure add further support to a causal relationship (Wood 1975; Fox 1992).

Diagnosis

The diagnosis of premature menopause is medically quite straight-forward and is easily understood by considering the ovary to be a typical hormone-secreting gland. The ovary is driven by two hormones, follicle-stimulating hormone (FSH) and luteinizing hormone (LH), made by the pituitary gland. The ovary in turn produces several hormones that control the release of LH and FSH in a feedback loop – oestrogen, inhibin and progesterone. If the ovary fails, the reduced supply of ovarian hormones is picked up by the pituitary gland, which makes more LH and FSH to 'push' the ovary harder. Ovary failure is diagnosed by measuring LH and FSH concentrations in the blood. In ovarian failure these are raised and the oestrogen concentration is reduced. The most sensitive of these hormones is the rise of FSH, which is the best early marker in premature menopause. Successful pregnancy is rare if the FSH measurement is twice normal (20 u/L instead of 10 u/L). In fact, FSH rises throughout the latter half of reproductive life in parallel with the reduced fertility that occurs after the age of 30 (MacNaughton et al. 1992).

The first sign of a premature menopause is usually when the periods stop. 'Amenorrhoea' describes the situation when no period has occurred for six months. 'Oligomenorrhoea' is when periods occur at intervals varying from 35 days to six months. A normal menstrual cycle may vary from 21-35 days. There are many reasons why periods stop, including pregnancy, weight loss and various hormone conditions. Some of the causes of amenorrhoea present-ing to the Middlesex Hospital are listed in Table 2.2 – a general practitioner would have a somewhat different list. Ovary failure is the only cause of amenorrhoea that produces the hormone picture of raised FSH and LH concentrations and reduced oestrogen. Along with amenorrhoea, the low oestrogen concentrations in the circulation lead to symptoms of flushing, mood change and vaginal dryness – these latter symptoms are common to some of the other causes of amenorrhoea and do not necessarily indicate a premature menopause.

Table 2.2: Causes of primary and secondary amenorrhoea in 660 women presenting to the Middlesex Hospital

	%
Polycystic ovary syndrome	34
Premature ovarian failure	27
Low body weight or excess exercise	11
Hypogonadotrophic hypogonadism	10
Hypopituitarism	4
Congenital abnormalities	1

In most instances when a 'menopausal picture' is found on hormone measurements, the diagnosis is secure and permanent. Occasionally, however, ovaries go through a temporary phase of low activity and subsequently return to normal life. For this reason, at least two hormone measurements taken some weeks apart are necessary before a definitive diagnosis can be made. Further, it may be useful to monitor FSH measurements over some months to establish a degree of variability of ovarian activity. Any attempts at infertility treatment might be focused on times in which the serum FSH concentration 'dips' into the normal range. Conversely, the witnessing of persistently raised FSH measurements may help some women come to terms with their diagnosis. As time passes it becomes less likely that the ovaries will return to activity, although rare cases of pregnancy occurring long after premature ovarian failure has been diagnosed have been reported. The mechanism of this return of function is a mystery and, frustratingly, no medical treatment seems to make it more likely.

Opinions vary as to whether biopsy of the ovaries is useful. Most doctors have abandoned biopsy in favour of ultrasound as a method of ascertaining the status of the ovaries. Ultrasound is able to detect ovaries in two thirds of women with premature ovarian failure, whereas in the days of ovary biopsy only 10–15% of women were thought to have a normal remnant of ovary tissue. At the time of writing, knowledge of the appearance of the ovary is somewhat academic as even the freshest-looking ovary cannot be made to work reliably by medical treatment if the FSH measurement is consistently raised. If and when immature eggs can be successfully nurtured in a test tube to allow fertilization, then knowledge of the appearance of the ovary will be important. At present, only mature eggs ready for ovulation can be used for in vitro fertilization (IVF) (see Chapter 9).

We routinely apply the following investigation in order to define the causes of premature menopause:

- Karyotype – high resolution chromosome analysis is particularly necessary for those presenting with primary amenorrhoea, but cytogenetic defects have been found in women with POF presenting as late as 35 years.
- Autoantibodies screen – thyroid, adrenal and ovarian antibodies provide a comprehensive picture of endocrine autoimmunity. Anti-ovarian antibodies are positive in only a small percentage of women with premature menopause, suggesting that in most instances this routine test is not sufficiently sensitive to be useful. Antibodies of the rheumatoid group may also be positive in women with premature menopause, but the significance of this finding is uncertain.
- Serial FSH measurements – as described above, this manoeuvre is useful to establish whether ovarian damage might fluctuate, as a guide to the possibility of remission. At present this exercise must be considered educational, as its efficacy in terms of predicting remission has not been demonstrated.
- Pelvic ultrasound – ovaries and follicles can be identified in approximately two-thirds of women with premature menopause (Conway et al. 1996). While this figure is encouraging, a positive ovarian ultrasound has poor predictive value for remission from POF. Conversely, we have yet to see remission when ovaries cannot be identified by an experienced ultrasonographer.

Prognosis

The process of the menopause, whether natural or premature, is variable in timing (Burger 1996). In some women, a completely regular menstrual cycle stops abruptly, never to return. In others, the transition from normal 'function' to the complete menopause takes several years of fluctuating ovarian activity. When the menopause transition is long and drawn out, the fluctuating hormone levels can be particularly disturbing. Rarely, ovarian damage appears to be partial but stable with no apparent progression to the complete menopause. This condition of raised serum FSH concentrations and infertility accounts for many women described as having ROS.

Once periods have ceased for six months and the diagnosis of premature menopause is secure, in our experience fewer than 1 in 100 women experience a return to fertility and achieve a pregnancy. Spontaneous pregnancy is never impossible but it is very unlikely. Several findings make the possibility of spontaneous pregnancy more likely – fluctuating FSH measurements, the ability to identify ovaries on ultrasound (Conway et al. 1996) and the association with autoimmunity or chemotherapy. Women who have identifiable autoimmune damage to the ovary or who have received anti-cancer treatments appear to be somewhat more likely to experience spontaneous remission. Thus clinics that focus on autoimmunity might quote a remission rate of up to 10%, while those taking a wider range of referrals might see only 1% remission.

The history of fertility treatments in women with premature menopause has been plagued by anecdotal reports of occasional successes, which, in retrospect, have usually been random events. Further, given the background fertility rate of 1–10%, only a large series would have the power to detect a real pro-fertility effect of any given treatment. It seems likely therefore, that new treatments will have to be subjected to a large multicentre randomized trial before they can be accepted as being genuinely effective. So the diagnosis of premature menopause must bring with it an expectation that fertility is only likely to be achieved through ovum donation and that oestrogen will need to be replaced on a long-term basis. Hormone replacement therapy probably has no effect on the chances of pregnancy; that is, if a miracle pregnancy is going to happen then HRT will not prevent it.

Young women who experience premature menopause not only have to face the prospect of infertility, but also have to consider years of oestrogen replacement treatment. The prognosis for those who do not take oestrogen is clear in some respects. Women with long-term oestrogen deficiency have a reduced risk of breast cancer and probably of thrombosis. These benefits have to be balanced against the increased risk of heart disease and osteoporosis. As heart disease and osteoporosis are far more common than breast cancer, it seems likely that the overall benefit of oestrogen replacement treatment is to improve not only the quality but also the duration of life. Decisions about HRT must be made, however, on an individual's balance of risk and benefit, and blanket policies can only form a guide to the process.

Future prospects

Premature menopause has long been neglected by medical research, with very few advances over the past 20 years. Suddenly much attention has been focused on the developing ovary and on possible assisted reproductive methods. Basic research is investigating the control of the destruction of eggs within the ovary. Further investigation of the genes involved in families with a history of premature menopause is another lead that may provide an insight into possible causes.

In the field of assisted reproduction, two possibilities are imminent. First, germ cells may be preserved at a very low temperature by means of cryopreservation (Newton et al. 1996). Frozen pieces of ovary tissue may be grafted back into the body once the threat to the ovary is over. The first partial success of ovarian autografting was reported in the press in October 1999. This form of treatment will be of importance only for women undergoing cancer treatment in whom permanent ovary damage is likely and in whom the starting point is normal ovarian function. A second and more technically challenging option is to mature primitive germ cells still present within the ovary. In vitro maturation of these ova to the point that would allow fertilization would be the goal. At present it is impossible to fertilize such primitive eggs and it is estimated that a breakthrough in this field is still many years away.

Chapter 3
Mid-life menopause: psychological and social meanings

Myra Hunter

The menopause literally means a woman's last menstrual period. This happens, on average, between the ages of 50 and 51, but, as pointed out throughout this book, with a wide age range. This definition suggests that the menopause happens overnight or at a single point in time. However, a woman's last menstrual period takes place after a gradual process of physiological change and its timing can be uncertain. For example, menstrual periods can stop and then restart again rather unpredictably (Kaufert & Gilbert 1988). The average duration of the menopause transition is estimated to be approximately four years, from the first menstrual cycle changes until 12 months after the last menstrual period, although again there is considerable variation (McKinlay et al. 1992a). Biological or bodily changes during the menopause transition occur at several levels and include hormonal changes (lowering of oestrogen levels and raised follicle-stimulating hormone, FSH), menstrual irregularity and cessation of periods, and, for many women, hot flushes and night sweats. Women's experience of these changes can vary considerably; for example, some have no experience of hormone changes or hot flushes.

In this chapter I aim to describe some of the varied psychological and social meanings of the menopause. For example, as well as meaning changes within the body, the menopause might also be seen as a marker of reproductive state, a threat to health, a stage of the life cycle, the onset of ageing or as a change of life. A woman's subjective experience of the menopause is therefore positioned between her perception of biological changes and the symbolic meanings or discursive constructions of the menopause. The aim is not to separate the body and mind and social influences but to see these as having a simultaneous and complex impact on experience. This perspective has been termed 'embodied subjectivity' (Rothfield 1997) or a material-discursive approach (see Ussher 1997b). In the context of the menopause, 'material' could refer to biological changes, such as the timing of the menopause (whether it happens in a woman's early forties or fifties), health problems, hot flushes and menstrual periods, and also to social and economic factors, such as experience of employment and social support. The 'discursive' element refers to the symbolic representations of menopause as a complex process involving varied bodily changes, the meaning of which are very much influenced by the material context and discursive constructions of gender, ageing and reproduction (Hunter & O'Dea 1997).

> There is no single discourse of menopause. Discussions of menopause may refer to biology or politics, hormones or feminism, psychoanalysis or social control, and when it comes to individual experiences, women provide widely varying accounts.
>
> (Komesaroff 1997)

In the following sections the development and impact of various meanings of the menopause are described. These are then discussed in relation to quantitative and qualitative studies of women's experience of 'on-time' menopause.

Menopause as madness

The association between a woman's reproductive body and her psychological wellbeing, and even her sanity, was perpetuated by psychoanalytic, psychiatric and gynaecological thinking in the nineteenth century. Expressions of distress or dissatisfaction could be interpreted as sexual or 'hysterical' in origin and gynaecological surgery was used as a treatment for insanity (Showalter 1987). Treatments suggested for 'symptoms' of the menopause were so unpleasant that they may well have deterred women from admitting any distress; for example, doctors introduced ice into the vagina and applied leeches to the labia and cervix.

Until 1980, when it was removed from the *Diagnostic and Statistical Manual of Mental Disorders* (DSM III) classification of psychiatric disorders, it was believed that the menopause was a cause of psychosis (involutional melancholia) (Krafft-Ebbing 1877). Psycho-analytic theories have tended to promote the view of the menopause as a neurosis and time of loss. At the menopause women become depressed because they mourn their loss of femininity and sexuality. A pessimistic picture was painted when this phase of life comes to an end:

> for reality has actually become poor in prospects, and resignation without compensation is often the only solution
>
> (Deutsch 1945)

Thus the end of reproductive life is expected to signal a morass of misery and an end to any sense of usefulness (Ussher 1989).

With the development of hormone replacement therapy (HRT), the treatment of menopausal women shifted from the domains of psychiatry and psychoanalysis to gynaecology and endocrinology. Instead of attributing sadness to loss of femininity and sexuality, a biological explanation is given – depression is caused by lowering or fluctuating hormone levels. The evidence concerning the relationship between depression and menopause is discussed in a later section in this chapter.

Menopause as change of life

'The change of life' in popular discourse reflects the view that the menopause might be paralleled by role changes and emotional and social adaptations that may occur during mid-life. It has been described as a period of adjustment, involving ending of the parental role, launching children into the adult world, reassessment of relationships, possible widowhood and loss of parents. While on average a woman who marries and has children in her twenties or early thirties may experience loss of parents and children leaving home in her late forties/early fifties, most women's lives do not conform to these traditional stages.

Children leaving home is not necessarily stressful and there is some evidence to suggest that women report more physical symptoms when young adults stay at home beyond expectations (Hunter 1992). However, women may experience bereavements for the first time during mid-life. Greene (1983) found that losses, including bereavements and loss of support through divorce or friends moving away, were the most potent predictors of distress in middle-aged women, especially for those who were already dealing with additional life stresses. Life stresses may occur during mid-life but, despite popular images, mid-life is generally not considered to be more stressful than other life stages, such as early motherhood (Boulet et al. 1985).

Menopause defining sexuality

Historically, female sexuality and reproductive potential have been seen as synonymous. For example, in the nineteenth century sexual arousal after menopause was considered highly undesirable and sexual intercourse potentially harmful. Tilt (1870) viewed sexual desire in a menopausal woman as a sign of 'morbid irritation' or 'uterine disease', requiring medical treatment. Symptoms of the menopause were often blamed on earlier sexual indiscretions, and the expression of sexual desire, or 'crises erotiques', by menopausal women was considered ludicrous or tragic.

In the twentieth century, hormonal treatments are seen as having the potential to restore sexual functioning in menopausal and older women. Therefore the earlier assumptions about reproductive potential and sexuality are maintained but can be overridden by medical practice. Here the woman's sexuality is positioned as being within her body. Thus the menopausal women can be seen as losing her sexuality but, at the same time, having it redeemed by medical treatment. Such discursive practices are likely to increase anxiety about sexuality. In fact, studies suggest that the menopause is not necessarily associated with changes in sexuality; some women report a decrease, others an increase, but the majority report no change in sexual activity and enjoyment (Gannon 1994). It is interesting that, in contrast to those applied to women, cultural stereotypes of sexuality in the ageing male reflect expectations of continuity, virility and potency.

Menopause as disease

While there is no direct record of the menopause in medical writing before the eighteenth century, there is indirect evidence of the 'treatment' of the menopause well before this. Views of menopause as a pathological state date back at least as far as Roman times, when menstrual blood was seen as poisonous. It was argued that after the cessation of menstruation, toxins previously excreted via menstruation were 'retained', destroying the body from within and causing physical, sexual and emotional decline. Blood letting, by cutting veins or applying leaches was a common treatment used to attempt to preserve wellbeing and physical and sexual attractiveness (Wilbush 1979).

Menopausal and climacteric complaints were first treated by doctors in eighteenth-century France. One of the early books was by Gardanne, who in 1816 was the first to use the term 'menespausie', which he later shortened to menopause. It was not until 1857 that a link was discovered between the functioning of the ovaries and the menopause. In the 1920s the main hormones produced by the ovaries were identified, and the first injections of oestrogens were attempted in Germany and the USA in the 1930s.

It is the biomedical discourse that dominates twentieth-century research literature and media accounts of the menopause. The menopause is seen as an oestrogen-deficiency disease, a cluster of physical and emotional symptoms that can be treated by HRT. An influential proponent of HRT, Robert Wilson (1966), in his book *Feminine Forever*, claimed that his 'youth pill' (oestrogen) could avert 26 psychological and physical complaints. 'Total femininity' could be preserved. The menopausal woman was depicted as 'an unstable oestrogen starved' woman who is responsible for 'untold misery of alcoholism, drug addiction, divorce and broken homes'. Although this position is now considered extreme, the view of menopause as a medical problem is still prevalent today.

The boundaries of the 'disease' have broadened over the past 20 years from a transitional state, in which women experienced hot flushes and night sweats, to a more permanent postmenopausal condition, rendering women prone to chronic health problems, such as osteoporosis and cardiovascular disease. Moreover, there has been a tendency in recent years to define menopausal women as a group with high health risks (Palmlund 1997). While increasing research interest into the health problems of older women, this perspective might implicitly suggest that the menopause is to be avoided (by HRT), since a host of problems might ensue if treatment is not sought. The broadening of the definition also implies that HRT should be used by the majority of women, even if they are not experiencing problems.

Media and pharmaceutical representations of the menopausal woman (taking HRT) currently present her as lively, energetic, healthy and physically attractive, thereby implying that, with medication, women can avoid the ageing process and can be in control of their health and their lives. The promotion of HRT places the menopause within a very medical discourse and plays on fears of ill-health and also on women's fears of ageing (Worcester &Whatley 1992). The medical model of the menopause at a discursive level is not to be confused with the reality of an individual women's experience. However, the two are intimately interlinked. How doctors view and treat women is influenced by the current medical model, and this model also determines how women are seen in the wider society, including how they interpret bodily changes and how they feel they are expected to look and behave (Kaufert & Lock 1997).

Menopause as a natural developmental phase

The sociocultural perspective on the menopause was developed in the 1970s by feminists, sociologists, anthropologists and others, partly in reaction to the growing predominance of the medical model. Here, menopause is viewed as a natural developmental process having little or no direct effect on women (see Kaufert 1982). Menopausal problems are seen as largely socially determined, being the result of negative stereotypes towards menopause and ageing, as well as women's limited social roles (Neugarten 1979; Parlee 1976). Sociological studies of attitudes to the menopause and experience of symptoms within and between cultures demonstrate the variability of 'menopausal symptoms' (Avis et al. 1993).

Cross-cultural studies provide many examples of how menopause can be a positive event, particularly when it signifies a change in social status (Davis 1986; Rice 1995). One of the first detailed anthropological studies was carried out by Marsha Flint, who talked to women of the Rajput caste in northern India about the menopause (Flint 1975). The menopause, she found, was accompanied by a marked change in status; Rajput women who no longer menstruated could emerge from purdah and enter public life. They became free to visit other households and to join in social gatherings. Not surprisingly, these women looked forward to this time of life and, when asked, reported no menopausal symptoms.

In general, women living in non-Western societies appear to

report fewer symptoms during the menopause compared with those living in Western societies (Payer 1991). For example, in Japan, symptoms characteristic of the menopause are headaches, dizziness and stiff shoulders; hot flushes and night sweats are experienced less frequently than in North America and cause less discomfort (Avis et al. 1993). As well as differences in attitudes and values, cultural practices can influence biological factors that in turn might shape a woman's experience of menopause. For example, Beyenne (1986) carried out a study in Mexico and in Greece and noted the material differences between cultures, such as diet, reproductive practices and exercise, which might, in addition to attitudes and values, explain the marked cultural variations in reports of menopausal experiences. Cross-cultural studies, however, also challenge the assumption that the menopause is something that can 'naturally' be experienced as either positive or negative. A person's body is the centre of ongoing dynamic interactions with physical, social and economic surroundings (Richters 1997). For further discussion of early menopause and ethnicity see Chapter 6.

Social scientists and feminist writers have critically examined Western assumptions about the menopause and have drawn attention to the negative effects of over-medicalization of the menopause. For example, the biomedical perspective can be seen as positioning women as deficient in relation to men and setting norms for what beliefs and actions are 'appropriate' for middle-aged women. Feminist writers have pointed to the need for women to have more balanced information about the menopause and more opportunities to talk about it in order to challenge stereotypic images of middle-aged women and practices that might pathologize and devalue older women.

Another perspective can be described as New Age or spiritual feminist, in which the potential power of the older women is acknowledged. Rituals or rites of passage have been developed to help women to harness their power and wisdom as they pass through the menopause (see Andrews 1993). The relatively recent construction of the menopause as a health problem has replaced a representation of the older woman as culturally approaching the status of an oracle, witch, healer, soothsayer, wise woman, harridan and virago (Campioni 1997). In a similar vein, Germaine Greer celebrates the opportunity to throw off cultural constraints of 'femininity' and to resist rigidly defined sex roles:

The climacteric marks the end of apologising. The chrysalis of conditioning has
once and for all to break and the female woman finally to emerge.

(Greer 1991)

Mid-life menopause: women's experiences

An examination of the discourses of menopause reveals the varied
and largely negative connotations that menopause has in many
cultures. These social meanings are likely to present women with an
additional task when facing menopause – how to deal with the
bodily or biological changes that occur, but also how to maintain
self-esteem when the social significance of these changes is negatively
connoted. As outlined above, social meanings can also provide
contradictory messages. For example, the biomedical and the socio-
cultural/feminist perspectives represent quite polarized positions
(Kaufert et al. 1992). I would argue that the biomedical view tends to
neglect social influences and, arguably, the sociocultural view has
traditionally ignored the body. A material-discursive or biopsychosocial model is needed to understand both the physical changes and
their social meanings (Hunter & O'Dea 1997).

Most psychological and sociological research on menopause has
drawn on epidemiological studies to address the questions relating to
whether or not women's experiences of menopause are consistent
with stereotypes. For example, do women become more depressed
during the menopause? Are there specific symptoms that affect
women and what proportions of women might experience these? Do
any positive changes happen?

Quantitative studies

In the 1980s several prospective studies (Matthews et al. 1990;
Oldenhave 1991; Holte 1992; Hunter 1992; Kaufert et al. 1992;
McKinlay et al. 1992a) were carried out in North America and
Europe. The studies included a cross-sectional phase, as well as
following women for between three and five years across the
menopause transition. Overall, few changes in emotional wellbeing
or mood were evident in these non-clinic samples (see Hunter 1996).
The results of these studies suggest that the menopause is not necessarily associated with emotional distress as might be expected from
the social meanings of menopause described above. Similarly, there is
no substantial evidence to support the view that psychiatric disorder

is more prevalent during the menopause (see Pearce et al. 1995). There were some changes in reports of sexual interest, but not overall satisfaction with sexual relationships. Reduced sexual interest was associated with many factors that might partly explain the association with menopause, such as age, marital satisfaction, partner's sexual functioning, ill health and stress. Women who have undergone oophorectomy (removal of the ovaries) without HRT may experience sexual and emotional sequelae in response to a rapid reduction of oestrogen and testosterone.

Hot flushes and night sweats increased during the menopause transition as expected, but the prevalence rates averaged around 50%–60% of menopausal women, lower than the commonly quoted 70%. There was some evidence of a slight increase in psychological symptoms in perimenopausal women who have hot flushes and night sweats and an association between length of perimenopause and mood, which can be explained by prolonged exposure to hot flushes and night sweats. Women who experienced chronic ill health, such as arthritis or thyroid problems, were also more likely to report depressed mood at this time. There was also some evidence from North American studies that women who had undergone hysterectomy reported more psychological distress than those who had not.

When asked, the majority of women reported relief from the cessation of menstruation and the possibility of pregnancy. However, a proportion expressed negative beliefs and expectations about the menopause beforehand. Such beliefs (that the menopause is associated with a host of physical and emotional problems) were found to predict depressed mood and other symptoms when these women reached the menopause (Hunter 1992). This finding provides evidence that social stereotypes about the menopause may in turn have a negative impact on women's experience of the menopause.

There was considerable variation between women in experience of the menopause and clearly some women do feel low or depressed during the menopause transition. Women who were depressed and those who experienced frequent hot flushes were most likely to seek medical help. Depressed mood was associated particularly with a history of depression, together with low socioeconomic status, not being employed outside the home and negative beliefs about the menopause (Hunter 1992). Psychological problems were associated with psychosocial factors to a greater extent than with stage of menopause.

Overall, epidemiological studies suggest that for the majority of women the menopause does not lead to changes in psychological symptoms, apart from possible secondary effects resulting from problematic hot flushes and night sweats. Taken together with cross-cultural findings, the notion of an essentially biological cause of distress is certainly challenged by recent research. Similarly, studies have failed to find an association between measures of depressed mood and hormone levels (oestradiol, progesterone, FSH and luteinizing hormone). Nevertheless, it remains possible that a rapid withdrawal of hormones might result in greater psychological distress. Treatment studies using HRT to improve mood have produced equivocal results. There is some evidence of a 'mental tonic' effect, i.e. an uplifting of mood, but little support for the use of HRT in the treatment of depression or psychological problems that may have a variety of causes (Hunter 1990; Pearce et al. 1995).

Qualitative studies

There have been few qualitative studies of how women themselves talk about or discursively construct the menopause. Those that have been published include descriptions of the pervasiveness of biomedical discourse (whether women's language reflected or resisted it) (Dickson 1990) or how medical discourse can function to enable some women to acknowledge distress and seek help (Daly 1995). In a study comparing women of different ages, Martin (1987) found that the vast majority of older women she interviewed saw the menopause in a positive light, while younger women tended to have a more negative view of the menopause.

In a recent study of women's accounts of mid-life menopause (see Hunter & O'Dea 1997), we used a qualitative methodology (thematic discourse analysis; Potter & Wetherell 1987), based on interviews with middle-aged women, to examine the ways in which the social meanings of menopause are reproduced in women's accounts. In particular, we were keen to explore how women talked about their experiences in the context of often negative, and potentially conflicting, discourses surrounding the menopause.

Forty-five women, aged 49 to 51 (from the age/sex register of a general practice in north London that served a large, socially mixed catchment area), responded to an invitation to talk to a researcher about their health, wellbeing and their lives. Fifty-six percent left school at the age of 16, while 44% continued education; 82% were married or cohabiting; and 75% described themselves as white-British. Fifty-one percent felt that they were currently going through the menopause, 16% were taking HRT, 20% were unsure as to their stage of menopause and 13% felt that they had not yet started it. The following analysis was based on the responses of the 37 women who saw themselves as menopausal, postmenopausal or who were taking HRT.

We used semi-structured interviews, which included open questions about their lives, their general health and the menopause. The interviews were tape recorded with the permission of participants and were transcribed verbatim. The texts and the tapes were repeatedly read and listened to by both authors and discussed. Six broad themes were identified from the women's accounts, and these are outlined briefly below. More than one theme was mentioned by a number of women.

Bodily changes

How women defined themselves in relation to the menopause tended to elicit discussion of physical changes, particularly hot flushes and night sweats. Menstrual and minor physical and emotional changes were mentioned, but to a lesser extent. Descriptions of hot flushes and night sweats varied considerably between women, many viewing them as not problematic:

> Maybe, about two years ago I was feeling hot at times, hot flushes but no more... It wasn't for long.

> I get hot at times but it doesn't bother me. If it's hot I just open the window but otherwise I don't have any ill effects at all.

However, several found them troublesome or embarrassing and there was a general concern about other people's reactions:

> The first time I got it I felt that everyone was looking at me; I used to go bright red and feel embarrassed. It only lasted a few minutes but does happen sometimes when I'm talking to people now: I feel uncomfortable. All the blood rushes to my face.

Hot flushes were also experienced as more problematic in certain situations, such as on the underground and when disrupted sleep affected ability to deal with work:

> You think hot flushes – poof nothing, easy peasy, but you can actually feel the sweat trickling down your head when you wake up during the night and then you're tired the next day, desperately because you can't sleep...and then you go to work and you're sat on the underground and because there's no movement of air, so it's drip, you want to take all your clothes off.

So the experience of hot flushes and night sweats is variable and partly influenced by the woman's social context and lifestyle.

Menopause as non-event: continuation of the self

The most commonly voiced theme was that the menopause had no or few consequences for the women at all. They tended to describe themselves as not particularly changed by the menopause:

> Nothing particular. I'm more concerned with getting on with the next week.

> Nothing really, it's part of life.

> It hasn't made me anything better or anything worse. I feel no different in myself.

Accounts of bodily changes were to some extent separated from how they felt the menopause had impacted upon themselves:

> I didn't like my periods being irregular or my body feeling different but in myself, well, I still felt that inside I hadn't changed.

> Physically it was nice not to have periods but that was counterbalanced by the sweats. Emotionally I was quite happy about it.

No more periods!

Cessation of menstruation was seen as a positive change by all the women who commented on menstrual changes. Menstruation was generally talked about as something negative and relief expressed about its absence:

> It's nice to get it over with and not have periods any more.

> I've never enjoyed having periods.

Relief was expressed particularly by women who had had heavy or problematic menstrual periods:

> I was a person who suffered an awful lot with my periods and it stopped me doing a lot of things when I was younger because I had such heavy periods and

now I can do anything I want. At one time if we planned to go away for the weekend and I had a period I was in such a state that I didn't want to go away.

Menopause as change in reproductive stage

While there was a general awareness that the menopause marked the end of a woman's reproductive phase of life, the majority did not express unhappiness about this. For the majority of these 50-year-olds, reproductive decisions tended to have been made earlier in their lives:

> I never really wanted to have children so it never really worried me in that way. I'll be quite pleased in some ways.

> It won't make any difference for me because I was sterilized at 38 and I won't feel that I can't have children any more because I've been quite happy not having children for the last 12 years.

However, again there was variability. For one woman fertility problems meant that within her culture she was not considered as a potential marriage partner:

> Being of Greek parents they used to try and organize your life and marry you off and I used to find that there was no way I could ever marry because I couldn't have children. That was the only thing that really upset me, not being able to get married and have children. The doctors might be able to do something about it now. It's a bit late now.

Most women challenged the view of the menopausal woman grieving loss of fertility, although particular circumstances (such as the earlier death of a child) and cultural influences also shaped the individual meaning of the menopause as a reproductive event. The age when menopause occurs is very likely to influence individual reactions to the meaning of menopause as a change of reproductive stage.

The menopause as a sign of ageing

The menopause was inextricably associated with age. Being 50 and menopause were used interchangeably. However, the majority challenged the view that menopause necessarily marks the beginning of old age:

> It doesn't make me feel older if that's what you mean.

> Getting old [laughs] but it doesn't bother me that much. I don't get hangups about it.

However, some women did voice concerns about ageing, about time running out and fears about being old.

> I think once the menopause is over you feel as though you're fast approaching retirement and it doesn't seen so very long now to being old. It's a bit frightening that it's only a few years away and there's still lots of things to do. I think in 10 years' time I'll be old.

However, a more positive discourse relating to age, voiced by several women, was of the menopause as a time for reflection:

> It brings home to you that perhaps you're in the last half of life. I think as a consequence of that I've sat and taken stock a little bit about life. You sit and think, where are we going from here, what do I want to do now? It's a time for a bit of reflection about where you're going over the next few years.

Social context was again an important influence on perceptions of ageing. One women worked with teenagers in an office:

> I've never looked at myself as being in my fifties but I find that I do feel it more now ... because I'm working with people that are 17, 18, and I feel older now. It suddenly makes you think, God I'm 50, where has my life gone? But before I never had these feelings at all. I don't know whether it's to do with the menopause or not or just your working environment.

There were also comments about the particular problems middle-aged women face in a society in which the 'ideal woman' (in contrast to men) has to both look and feel young to be valued:

> I think it's awful. I don't think it's fair that women should have this at all but there you are. I still think that after 50, it's very hard for a woman. Men have the advantage. Generally speaking it's much harder over 50 for a woman to be young in her mind as well as how she looks.

Staving off the unknown: menopause as unspoken taboo

Although the interviewer used the word menopause, the women tended not to. 'It' and 'this' were used, suggesting that the menopause was not commonly discussed directly.

Similarly, women frequently talked about the menopause as if it was something that was happening but they were attempting to not face or trying to avoid. They talked about keeping busy, not thinking about it and not letting themselves go:

You have to put yourself in order as well because when you go through something like that you become like you are not interested in yourself ... like you want
to let yourself go. You have to occupy your mind. So I think for some women
who have nothing to do it must be really terrible for them. They must sit down
and think about it and become depressed.

I'm too busy to worry, I really don't think about it a lot.

Implicit in several accounts was the idea that if they did stop to find
out what 'it' was, there would be negative consequences. Others
voiced fears of something vague, difficult and non-specific happening to them, which was difficult to name or talk about, although
concerns about 'letting yourself go', 'becoming depressed' and losing
control were indirectly mentioned.

Two women described how by taking HRT they wiped out or
'staved off' the menopause for the time being:

Now it's wiped out, it's a non-event.

Well I feel OK about it, it's what other people desire and need from me that's the
difficulty. I've staved off the menopause until my husband catches up with me.

This woman had a young family and a younger husband and felt
that going through the menopause did not fit with her current life.

In this qualitative study, women's experience of mid-life
menopause was varied, multidimensional and influenced by social
context. Medical terminology was used when women initially
defined themselves in relation to the menopause (in terms of bodily
changes), but less so when they talked about the impact of the
menopause on themselves. In general, the women described the
menopause as having little overall impact, they talked of continuation of the self and relief from menstruation; for these women reproductive decisions, on the whole, were faced earlier in their lives.
Their accounts of the impact of the menopause were complex, varying with material circumstances, for example, working environment,
hot flushes, past pregnancies and heavy periods.

Women can face a considerable discursive task at the menopause
– to maintain a positive sense of self amidst menopause and age
changes which are unduly negatively connoted. The majority of the
women we spoke to did this by describing menopause as having little
impact on themselves, being pleased to be free from periods and

unaffected by not being able to have children. While women challenged assumptions based on biomedical and psychoanalytical theories, they did so by positioning themselves in relation to these discourses. For example, by saying the end of the reproductive life stage is not a problem, or the menopause did not produce symptoms. Other ways of negotiating negative images of menopause was to see other women as being more prone to problems and by avoiding or staving off the menopause, for example, by keeping busy or taking HRT.

I would argue that fears engendered by negative social meanings were difficult to talk about directly and tended to be avoided in a variety of ways. By 'staving off' the menopause some women did not have the opportunity of finding out whether their experience would in fact conform to their image; in this way taboos about menopause are easily maintained. A similar process has been described by Rich (1992) in relation to the maintenance of ageist attitudes:

> Given the hazards of passing and the fact that so many old people themselves have lived a lifetime of fear, contempt and patronizing of the old, it is easy to see why most old people share with other members of society the stereotyped view of old people and also refuse to define themselves as old.

Conclusions

The menopause is a vague and broad term which has multiple social and historical meanings. For women experiencing 'mid-life menopause', the results of quantitative and qualitative studies provide some reassurance that, despite the stereotypic views of the menopausal women as mad, diseased or in decline, the majority do come through the menopause transition without it having major impact on their lives, and some welcome the end of menstruation. They do, however, have to deal with uncertainties, discrimination and fears, which are engendered by unhelpful social discourses, particularly relating to gender and ageing. As well as factors such as experience of hot flushes, life stresses and ill-health, the timing of the menopause is likely to have a major impact on the experience of menopause. For women with early menopause the task of negotiating bodily changes and social meanings is likely to be more problematic. Bodily changes may well have a more profound impact; for example, the meaning of cessation of menstruation, hot flushes and infertility are likely to be different for women experiencing premature menopause. Nevertheless, it is important that myths about mid-life menopause are challenged so that younger women can approach this stage of life with balanced information and realistic expectations about what might happen, and so that the self-esteem of women who do experience early menopause is not diminished further by the internalization of images of menopause that emphasize decline, ageing and psychological ill-health.

To demystify the menopause it might be beneficial to promote a language that is more specific and which discriminates between different aspects of the process. For example, the women interviewed in the qualitative study above talked about and evaluated hot flushes, menstrual and reproductive changes quite differently. Several women commented that the menopause is still a taboo and that few opportunities exist at this stage of life to discuss feelings and experiences in depth. Clearly, changes are needed at social, political and individual levels. For example, health education about the menopause could be offered in schools and in the workplace; representations of middle-aged and older women in the media could be increased to reflect a range of experiences and lifestyles. In a clinical setting, I work with groups of middle-aged women in order to provide a place for discussion about social and cultural meanings of the menopause and to examine their impact on experience of this stage of life (Hunter & Liao 1995; Liao & Hunter 1994). (For further discussion of group approaches, see Chapter 11.) Such groups might help to develop common understandings, to acknowledge differences between women, and to reinforce the sense of agency and resistance to stereotyped images that the middle-aged women in the qualitative study described in this chapter clearly voiced in their personal accounts.

Part 2
The experience

Chapter 4
The experience

DANI SINGER

> My ordeal with premature menopause started almost two years ago...if only I had recognized those symptoms for what they were, things might have been different. But ... out of my desperate attempt to feel normal again, I consented to have a total hysterectomy. I was 32.
>
> (Molly 1993)

A premature menopause for Molly constituted a 'crisis' and 'ordeal' in which she felt completely alone. This chapter considers responses to premature menopause from the perspective of women themselves.

In 1996, I carried out a research study to find out how women experienced premature menopause, what were their main concerns and how they dealt with the changes in their lives (Singer 1996). I was also interested in looking at how women who have undergone a premature menopause maintain a sense of self and identity in the face of potentially negative social meanings relating to menopause. In an attempt to understand the complexities involved, the study included 13 women and focused on the detailed 'stories' of particular women in specific situations while searching for patterns across them (Smith et al. 1995).

A qualitative methodology was used to analyse themes in women's descriptions of premature menopause. This was broadly based on the thematic discourse analysis technique of Potter & Wetherell (1987). The interest was primarily in examining how, in their individual accounts, women described the impact of premature menopause and their attempts at maintaining self-esteem in the face of the multiple dilemmas raised. Semi-structured interviews were conducted, each approximately one and a half hours long (Merton et al. 1990). Interviews were conducted in a conversational manner and in a relaxed atmosphere, usually in the woman's home. Confidentiality was assured and interviews were audiotaped with the woman's permission. Analysis involved listening to the tapes, reading and rereading the transcripts and peer group discussion to draw out broad themes. For a more detailed discussion of methodology and analysis, see Singer & Hunter (1999).

The mean age of the 13 participants at time of interview was 31, with ages ranging from 23 to 46 years (Table 4.1). The mean age at menopause was either 28 (according to the women's own diagnosis) or 29 (based on medical definition). One of the 13 women, had had a surgical menopause, another's was the result of radiation treatment. Premature menopause often took time to be diagnosed. Frequently there was a gap, occasionally of several years, between the women's own sense of something being amiss and the medical confirmation of it.

Table 4.1: Profile of women diagnosed with premature menopause

Age in 1996	Age at menopause	Age periods stopped	Marital status	Number of children	Additional health issues	Menopausal treatment
40	30	30	single	0	-	none
37	34	34	divorced (+ partner)	3	-	HRT
38	32	28	single (+ partner)	0	underactive thyroid	HRT*
28	27	27	single	0	tumour (radiotherapy treatment)	HRT
38	35	35	divorced (+ partner)	1	-	(HRT) declined
23	18	16	single (+ partner)	0	-	contraceptive pill
41	38	35	divorced (+ partner)	1	overactive thyroid	HRT*
36	34	34	married	2	hysterectomy	HRT
41	25	24	married	2 (adopted)	-	HRT
42	40	37	single	0	lupus	HRT*
38	33	22	married	1	-	(HRT) declined
36	30	22	married	1	endometriosis	HRT
46	40	40	married	1	-	HRT

*Indicates additional medication.

With the exception of one Asian woman, all participants were white. Eight were educated to degree level and all worked at least part time. Just under half were single and of these most were in heterosexual relationships at the time of interview. Just over half were or had been married or lived with partners. Of these, several had children and in one case had adopted children. Among the women with no children, one was actively seeking partial custody of her ex-partner's child.

Several broad themes emerged from the women's accounts:

- initial reactions to physical changes
- impact of diagnosis
- communication with health professionals
- impact of infertility
- premature menopause as early ageing
- personal identity and social relationships.

These are presented below.

Initial reactions to bodily changes

Nearly universal for the participants in this study was confusion about what was happening to their bodies:

> You're having all these symptoms and you don't know what's wrong with you. Once you can categorize it, it provides perspective. When I had hot flushes, first they said I had an internal infection, then different specialists said different things. Some said 'menopause', some said 'no' – but if it's not menopause, then what's wrong with me?

For anyone who feels they are deviating from the norm, etiology is likely to be an important concern. While some women in this study appeared upset about their inability to produce children, others worried about the effects on long-term health. Efforts were made to find positive compensations, but mainly there was considerable anxiety and distress around not being like other 'real' women and, worst of all, a feeling of being 'so awfuly alone'.

During the interviews, women seemed to find talking about their physical symptoms a way of easing into a more intimate discussion of what their experience meant to them. They talked primarily about stopped or missed periods, hot flushes and other 'classic' menopausal symptoms, which, sooner or later, had been medically confirmed. A few had experienced such symptoms, but did not make the connection with menopause:

> Hot flushes, missed periods – naturally I presumed I was pregnant.

> I started getting palpitations and those infamous flushes, which I'd heard and read about, but it didn't occur to me that this is what it is.

For others they were very frightening:

> The first time was missed heart beats and palpitations – terrifying. I really thought I was dying, they were so severe.

The language used to describe the bodily changes was often emotive:

> Sticky, heavy disgusting periods.

> I couldn't bear anyone to touch me. I would suddenly get this disgusting feeling – it sort of starts from inside, you know it's happening and there's nothing you can do about it and you feel like you're dripping buckets.

At times the physical manifestations of menopause were particularly hard to bear as they seemed to invite unwanted attention:

> It's like somebody's got a hot water bottle round your neck – the heat rises and you feel like a beacon.

Several words cropped up repeatedly: 'obviously', '(bloody) freak', 'abnormal' and 'not natural', implying a painful sense of feeling different from others. Most hardly used the word 'menopause', preferring to call it 'it', or referred to it in obliquely ('have it', 'got it', 'gone through it'), although there was also evidence of a desire to speak out:

> Sometimes I want to shout it out in the college bar: 'Look for God's sake, be a bit nicer to me, (laugh) – I can't have children'.

Finding the appropriate words was often described as problematic, and there was evidence of a marked reluctance to be labelled menopausal. When discussing how they explained their premature menopause to others, several women indicated that they preferred to talk of 'hormonal imbalance' or 'infertility', or preferably, say nothing at all:

> I always worry about how people will react. I'm quite cool about telling people about my tumour, but with the menopause, I feel embarrassed.

I've just said: 'Oh, there are problems' or 'the ovaries aren't working properly', which is true, but doesn't have the finality of what actually happened.

It's too difficult – I just sort of brush it off and say 'we don't want any'.

Embarrassment at disclosing her menopause led one woman to conclude, in relation to job applications:

I'll just say I don't want children. It's terrible when you have to lie. But if you say you're menopausal, you're not quite 100%: not 100% healthy, not 100% in your mind; you're (perceived as) emotional, irrational.

Only one woman used menopause as an active verb, almost as an act of defiance:

I'm glad I menopaused. It may have been early, but it's been normal.

The feminist idea that if the shoe was on the other body so to speak, and men menstruated, it would become an 'enviable, boast-worthy event' (Steinem 1981) was echoed by a number of women:

If men went through the menopause, I don't think we'd be fobbed off as much.

If men went through it, there'd be answers.

Although negative consequences were dominant in the women's accounts, participants did talk about a few positive aspects of a premature menopause – no more periods:

They were an inconvenience, more unpleasant and messy than painful or anything like that – and the expense, damn it!

It's bloody unfortunate that with HRT you get a bleed every month (laugh). I'd love to never bleed, but I don't want to get cancer, and hot flushes is a small price to pay.

Impact of diagnosis

On confirmation of the diagnosis, most of the women felt completely isolated, as the majority had never heard of this happening to anyone so young before. Words like 'shocking', 'devastating' and 'gutting' were used repeatedly. Some women described the impact of diagnosis as devastating:

It was almost like a death verdict. I remember being blasted with it, utterly shattered.

I went to the loo and cried for ages and ages. Then I saw my friend and cried a lot more and for the rest of the day.

Occasionally there was relief at finally knowing that what they were experiencing had a medical name:

When I have depressions, they're almost easier to deal with now, because there's a reason.

I was just so relieved, I could come to work and say, 'I'm sorry', I'd been under-performing or was so tired or had time off sick because of this – and they were as pleased as I am that it's sorted.

How negatively a diagnosis of premature menopause was viewed depended partly on whether either they themselves or those dear to them had experienced 'worse' losses:

It is a terrible thing to hear, but at least it came on top of 'you're not dying'. I suspect someone who hadn't had that would be so much more shocked than I was, who had time to prepare herself.

I wish it hadn't happened. What keeps me in check and puts me back in reality, is that I could have died. There was a 50–50 chance my tumour could have been malignant. If it had been, I'd be dead by now.

Most women expressed 'upset' at learning that they were experiencing an unexpected menopause. They talked of a lack of warning, a dearth of explicit information and the absence of practical advice on how to ameliorate and come to terms with what they were experiencing. This differed markedly from findings among 'on time' women, who tend to view menopause less uniformly. In this study, the narrow range of responses to a premature menopause, clustering on the negative end, was striking and seemed to hold regardless of individual circumstance. This response appeared to be aggravated by the experience of uncertainty, confusion and delay in diagnosis:

It was the normal shock: no, I don't believe this, they've already told me I'm not. Then very angry because I had to wait years for confirmation, then very depressed.

I didn't believe it. I thought, no, no, it must be something else, because of being much younger.

After I'd had anger, I got upset, because I thought: 'My God, I can't have children' – this plan that when I was more grown up (laugh) I'd have children. Eventually, I kind of accepted it.

Others reported that their discomfort was magnified by their doctor's response:

> I said, I think I'm going through menopause. They'd look at my age, they'd look at me, and say, 'No, it can't be, you're too young.' That was the response I got.

Sometimes premature menopause resulted in confusion about one's place in the generation table:

> I rang my mum up and said: 'This could mean that I'm your sister rather than your daughter.'

A distinction emerged between immediate reactions and long-term implications. Initially, nearly all women seemed to undergo a process of shock, anger, mourning and varying degrees of adjustment. A general consensus that a bereavement had occurred was evident. Grieving did not appear to follow a sequence of stages (Kubler-Ross 1970; Parkes 1972), but showed a fluid pattern of setbacks, ups and downs, to be worked through to assimilate what had happened.

Long-term implications varied according to both the current age of the women and their present circumstances. A premature menopause led a majority to realize that they could no longer take their health for granted. Many worried about their future health, physical and psychological:

> My bones are what I worry about.

> I'm scared that when my friends start having children, it'll freak me out a lot more than I think it's going to. A lot of times I think I'm really sorted, but at other times I'm really not at all.

Medically, the majority of women in this study underwent a premature menopause without any obvious precipitating factors, although a number did have additional health problems such as thyroid conditions, cancer or heart problems. Nevertheless, a large proportion believed they had 'done it' to themselves:

> It was my fault, I was to blame somehow. When I realized I couldn't (have a sexual relationship with a particular man when she was 24), just to please my mother, that it wasn't fair – that was the point where my body seemed to stop.

> I was working till the last minute and very fit. And then this birth, which was so awful. It's as if my body decided to give up after this trauma. It was so bad that something in me decided it had had enough.

People who know me incredibly well said I did it to myself, because I used to loathe contraception; really, really, loathe it.

Some attributed their premature menopause to hormonal factors:

I took the contraceptive pill from 18 to 22 and it was when I stopped that I had strange goings on with my periods.

A mixture of both the medical reasons they had been given and their own explanations were also put forward:

I understand enough about autoimmune diseases to understand that when your immune system is oversensitive, it attacks a part of your body it wouldn't usually. But the reason it happens is emotional.

Attributions could be more general:

It's just the lifestyle – we're on the go all the time. Most of us go out to work and raise a family, trying to fit everything in.

Several women resisted the stereotypical notion that the symptoms of menopause are 'all in your mind':

I've been told over and over until quite recently, that everything's that's wrong with me must be in my mind. They seem to treat 'mental pausal' women as if they are one, mental; two, diseased.

Although one or two did seriously worry about their sanity:

I thought I had a mental illness, because I was really nasty, a nasty piece of work.

Communication with health professionals

The women in the study felt that an essential aspect of health had been lost. Almost all accepted their condition as needing medical consultation, information, advice and treatment. Where children were desired, dependency on medical technology and expertise increased.

Physicians were consistently described as underestimating the distress caused by the enormity of the diagnosis. This is in keeping with earlier studies (Ley 1982). Almost all women had a vivid recall of what was said to them, often recounting it verbatim, thereby revealing the extent of the emotional impact. Usually only their bodies were discussed, leaving them feeling unseen and unheard as whole people:

> They don't tell you anything. They are not interested. They don't seem to have the time. It was just: 'Right, you're menopausal. Take this.'

Virtually all the women in the study heard judgements around failure and abnormality during their consultations with health professionals. Most were as affected by the manner of the telling as by its content. Nearly all spoke of the difficulties of obtaining adequate medical advice and being given wrong or incomplete information, often in a casual manner. Several mentioned premature and incorrect diagnosis. Sometimes the results were telephoned to them at work:

> The way he told me was very off-hand. He said: 'Oh, by the way, there might be some fall out.'

> The doctor was quite insensitive. There was no feeling of my emotional taking of it. It was just: 'this is the diagnosis'. And when I started crying, he just said: 'What are you crying about? You're not going to die.'

> They could have said it in a nice way. I just walked out of the clinic, reduced to tears. I still remember that doctor – I'd kill him if I saw him now, he upset me so much.

The way the diagnosis was communicated had important implications for how women received it:

> He glanced at my notes and said, 'You've had your menopause. My God, do you know how rare that is?' Well, I just looked at him and burst out laughing. I said, 'I know you're trying to be kind, but have you any idea how horrible that sounds? That makes me feel like an absolute bloody freak!'

Several had to work hard at convincing their doctors that what they were going through was real:

> They thought I was a hypochondriac.

> It's taken me years to convince them that there was something else besides neurosis.

The health professionals encountered by the women in this study were frequently described as being not only insensitive, but also unfamiliar with premature menopause. This served to heighten the woman's sense of isolation and her fears of being abnormal and not understood. Lack of knowledge often fed on shaky self-esteem, leading to a marked tendency to blame oneself:

> Nothing prepared me – so I felt very devastated and ashamed.

The majority of participants had been prescribed hormone replacement therapy (HRT). Women's reactions to HRT were generally positive, although there was concern about side effects. Most of the reasons put forward for taking HRT were to prevent osteoporosis, and to control hot flushes and mood swings. Some found HRT helpful in relieving symptoms and in improving their sense of wellbeing:

> I felt like a new person. I didn't feel tired, I could do more. I had loads more energy, I was sleeping better and the palpitations stopped.

> Obviously I'm on HRT. I went for a bone scan and it's terrific. I didn't believe it was going to make that much difference, but you're talking about high single figure percentage improvement in bone density, which is extraordinary.

One woman felt HRT made her premature menopause virtually a non-happening:

> All the symptoms disappeared. It was like a miracle, I was reborn – amazing. I've been told I have to have this oestrogen until I'm 60 or so – another 25 years. It's a long time to be relying on tablets, but if that's what's going to keep me going...

Perhaps not surprising, given the frequent controversies surrounding HRT, some women expressed ambivalence around its use.

> I struggled with that for a long time – should I, shouldn't I? All the things that 50-plus-year-old women think about, but I'd be on it a hell of a lot longer, 30–40 years.

> I don't know what HRT would do. It might not do any harm, but over a long period – I don't think you should put something in your body if you don't need it.

A few preferred to explore non-medical approaches:

> I'm more into natural methods like homeopathy. HRT made me very bloated. I put on over a stone – the only advantage was it made my skin better, but it didn't make me any happier.

Overall, HRT-induced bleeds were greeted with mixed feelings.

Some women expressed annoyance that the only benefit of menopause was taken away, while others felt them to be a normalizing influence:

> It made me feel more normal, even though they were brought on by drugs. Emotionally that makes me feel better, makes me feel a woman.

> There's something reassuring about having people seeing I have a box of tampons in the bathroom.

Impact of infertility

Infertility was the single most distressing aspect of a premature menopause described by the participants in this study, whether or not a woman already had children. This confirmed a previous study which demonstrated that over half (54%) of prematurely menopausal women with children experienced loss of fertility as disturbing (Baber et al. 1991).

Several participants expressed an intense yearning for the intimacy of the mother–baby relationship. In some instances, its loss led to a sense of isolation, as if a death had occurred. Among some of the women without children, the longed for relationship to the baby tended to be idealized.

> I love babies, if I could have one tomorrow I would. The best time of my life was when my children were babies. I like the fact that they were relying on me.

Most common was a sense of puzzlement at feeling punished while having done nothing wrong.

Being fertile was usually linked to the idea of being or becoming whole, leaving many of the women feeling 'incomplete' and so of less value. 'Robbed' of the fundamental power to create, some felt bereft of almost all power. Loss of reproductive capacity seemed aggravated by a fear of having to account publicly for this condition. Many viewed themselves as separated from their former selves, thrust into an uncomfortable time warp – a disjuncture also experienced in relation to body image, sexuality and ageing. Generally it was felt, although to varying degrees, that a 'complete' woman is one who is at least potentially fertile:

> I didn't feel like a 'real woman', I felt inferior.

> I can rationalize it, but it's sad, I can never have a baby that comes from me. That's terrible – it depresses me more than anything.

Several referred to the loss of the ability to bear children as a bereavement:

> Obviously the major loss is the fact that you can't have children. Even though after Jo, we decided not to have any more, deep down, I thought: 'Perhaps it will still happen.'

> I'm quite happy to have one (child) but (cries)...I just put it (having any more) into the back of my mind.

> Finally I realized I hadn't dealt with the feeling of loss: while I dealt with the practical side of things, emotionally I was probably crippling myself.

Occasionally women felt that they might be driven into dangerous behaviour by the intensity of their feelings:

> I just wanted to go and kill myself – when I'd be driving, I'd want crash into something. I almost did it, but then we decided to adopt a baby, and the thought of having a baby stopped me.

A minority managed to resist the notion that infertility bore any relationship to self-worth:

> The attitude that you can't be of any use apart from bearing children, that that's what you're put here for, is quite an insult.

In retrospect, the majority of participants expressed mixed feelings:

> When you're menopausal that's when you're not going to have children any more. Providing you're fit and well I don't see that as a problem ... On the other hand, I love babies. If I could have one tomorrow I would. The best time of my life was when my (three) children were babies, relying on me.

> I'm glad I menopaused, but it would have been impossible not to have a child. I had to have a child.

Several of the women felt that their choice had been unjustly curtailed or that they were left with only artificial and second-best choices (egg donation):

> Logically, I wouldn't have wanted another baby, two are a handful. But it's that the choice has been taken away.

> I've been robbed of a choice I might have had and would have wanted to have, had I been able to.

> I just wanted to have a child. I felt cheated, cheated by life, cheated by my body.

> Sometimes I think that's too unnatural, that's wrong and horrible. All the tests, the operations – I don't know.

Some rejected the offer of fertility treatment outright:

> I don't want to be anyone's guinea pig. I don't want to go through every month building myself up and crushing myself down again.

Just under half expressed a conscious or implied jealousy of, or anger at, others with children:

> Knowing that I won't have any myself, I get very angry when I see people mistreating children.

> Whenever I saw a mother and child on the street – every time, not just once in a while but every time – it reduced me to tears.

> I've got friends the same age as me having babies and it's strange. If they're boys, I think that's nice and go out and buy things for them. But my cousin just had a baby girl, and it was dreadful. She brought her over, and I didn't want to give her back. You have that longing. [Has two sons]

> When they have the first child I can be generous, but the moment they have a second, I get into this horrific sort of jealousy. [Has one child]

Although this was by no means always the case:

> Sometimes when I see my brother's children, I think: 'Thank God I don't have to deal with this.'

A theme which regularly appeared was that of a lost life plan or dreams. The majority of women automatically assumed they would have children. It was unclear whether the loss of this 'plan' was a loss primarily to themselves or of what they had taken on as part and parcel of being female in contemporary society:

> I'd always felt, like most girls growing up, that at some stage I'd probably have children. I know not all do, but I think the majority would, and I thought it would be me at some time.

> It was the one thing I really wanted. That's why we got married early, to start a family as soon as possible.

One or two saw a need to readjust previously held plans:

> You do have to make a conscious change. The lifestyle you had in the back of your mind is gone and you have to accept that.

However, there were also variations in views about motherhood:

> I've made my own life as an independent person, and it doesn't worry me that I

haven't got any. I'm not particularly maternal. [Single, no child]

I never was particularly motherly or desperately wanted children. [Married, mother of one]

Infertility led some women to shift where they placed their energies. Some responded by adopting children or actively contemplating it, yet others redirected their efforts into professional activities. Overall, an attitude of taking stock of their lives was common:

Practically, I have a different attitude towards work, now I know I'm going to be there until I'm 60 or 65.

I had to re-evaluate my position in the world, not take it for granted.

Some decided to devote more time to the children they did have in an attempt to get the most of life:

It's made me more determined to enjoy my life, also because of the shock – what else is round the corner for me?

Whether or not they already had a child, adopted or remained child-free, self-esteem could be deeply affected:

It was really awful, nobody understands. Everyone thinks you're silly when you cry every minute.

It's the pain and shame of being inadequate.

Since my diagnosis I've married, adopted two children so that side of my life is very stable and fine. But as for my own feelings about myself – there's something lacking in me, I'm not quite the person I should be.

Premature menopause as early ageing

Youth and fertility tend to be equated for women in a way they are not for men (Ussher 1992). This was evident in the majority of accounts by respondents who expressed dread at the prospect of wrinkling, fears of becoming 'ancient overnight' and the terror of being helpless to prevent it. The dream of perpetual youth had seemingly been extinguished. Being other than 'ideal' (young, fertile and attractive) as a woman had to be confronted:

Being feminine is definitely being young and having lots of energy. It's the age-old story: a man gets old and becomes more mature, a woman gets old and becomes an old hag.

On the whole, premature menopause seemed to draw women's attention to the ageing process and their own vulnerability and mortality. Because it felt so precipitous, several found it difficult to accept with equanimity:

> Absolutely gutting to discover that you've got the potential in 5–10 years' time to have osteoporosis. That was probably one of the most difficult things to deal with: you look at yourself in the mirror and say how can that be? I've always had a reasonable diet, got the right vitamins. To discover something like this is probably the most horrible thing, because it's something you really can't do anything about.

> It's having to accept that I am officially old no matter what my physical appearance may be – and that I'm on the downhill side, no ifs ands or buts about it.

When the association with ageing was triggered by a doctor's remarks, this could be especially disturbing:

> He was denying that I could have had it (menopause) because had I had one, I'd be wrinkled and old-looking. And I was thinking, I've been told, how could it not be true? And if it's true, am I suddenly going to sprout wrinkles?

It could be particularly worrying among women who were considerably older than their partners:

> There was an element of fear, because he is so much younger than me. I suddenly thought: 'My body's going to disintegrate – he won't desire me or love me any more. Maybe he wants more children, maybe...' – all those things.

However, some women attempted to resist the link between premature menopause and ageing:

> I don't think it's going to be a significant factor in ageing: going grey is going to be more significant.

> I don't feel any older. The brochures made you feel older.

The fear of premature ageing tended to exacerbate anxiety about being abnormal:

> It's because it's not the norm. Most people say: 'At my age', 'I'm at that age', and I think, 'Well, I'm not, not at all, I'm half the age.' My mum's going through menopause.

> There is a bit of a feeling of abnormality – horrible word. It's perfectly normal, just a funny age (laughs).

Several related this to a sense of unreality underscored by the lack of visible signs on their body. Looking in the mirror was often mentioned as a way of seeing if their condition 'showed' or leaked out in some way. Feelings ranged from being 'unrecognizable' to 'paranoid' about being old, or believing that her endocrinological age (the age of her internal organs) must be reflected in her mirror image. Even so, whether or not a premature menopause constituted something pathological did not go unchallenged:

> It's just something people go through. Unfortunately I went through it sooner than most.

The best that could be said for it was that one might get over it more quickly:

> Maybe I'll turn around when all my friends are 50 and go, 'Ha, ha, ha (laugh), been there, done that', I don't know.

As women approached the 'normal' age at menopause, there was relief that the discrepancy would diminish:

> It'll be easier once I'm at the age where it's expected.

Personal identity and social relationships

A premature menopause is a physiological process with profound implications for a woman's sense of self. It is also an event demarcating an 'I' that was before from the 'I' that is after menopause:

> You have to redefine yourself: suddenly you're somebody completely different.
>
> You think, this is the end of my life as I know it.

Occasionally women fell into extreme despair:

> I used to feel terrible, suicidal, because I felt I was nothing.

Usually, it was a matter of time before more positive feelings emerged:

> It took a while before I realized I hadn't really changed. I still looked the same. I hadn't turned into that little grey old lady overnight. As a matter of fact, I felt like doing more things.

With a premature menopause the 'self' as omnipotent creator of possibilities seemed to collapse. There may be fear of losing partners, the result of associating the menopause with the end of sexual life (Bertrand-Servais et al. 1993). Already feeling inadequate and embarrassed at not being picture-perfect in other ways, being unable to reproduce doubled the blow by barring the prematurely menopausal woman from being able to do what women 'should' be able to do – a concern often reflected in worries about being feminine and attractive, and having a 'good' body size and image.

Several participants felt their own sexuality, sexual desires and their desirability for others threatened:

> It's much more subdued – as if my body doesn't take it that seriously any more.

> Sometimes it makes me feel less sexy. I feel neutered, like my cat.

> How I relate to people is completely different. I'd be incapable of being flirtatious now, whereas that was my line before, definitely. I could get people to jump through hoops for me.

At 25, the youngest participant was particularly concerned about her sexual attractiveness and wondered how this might endanger prospective long-term relationships to men:

> It's made sex more problematic for me, although in some ways I think of it as less serious, because this happened before I went into sexual relationships. I've never had the scare of being pregnant from sex.

A few claimed to have lost all interest in sex:

> ...which makes it even harder to conceive, so it feels like a vicious circle.

Occasionally the view that they were no longer the same was resisted:

> It's not going to change me.

> I don't feel I'm losing any feminine side. I'm still me. It's more the health aspects that bother me.

Premature menopause was described by a number of the participants of this study as the start of mistrusting their bodies, affecting intimate, familial and social relationships. It is not only what happens inside her body that affects a woman, but what it means to her in her social context. In most cases, feeling no longer a 'real' woman was reflected in a strong concern with appearance:

> I felt I must look strange – it's the body being separate from the rest of you.
>
> I suddenly realized, I don't feel attractive. I felt terrible, like everyone was better than me.

The invisibility of premature menopause seemed to make it simultaneously easier and harder to bear. On the one hand, it made it more difficult to receive acknowledgement of the losses involved, thereby increasing a sense of vulnerability and isolation:

> If you're minus a hand, or you have a patch over your eye, or if you can't hear, these are all visible signs – people can make allowances, or sympathize, or help, but [with this] people forget you're susceptible to certain comments, that certain things still hit home.

On the other hand, it might mean that one could somehow 'get away' with it:

> You don't have a label saying 'my ovaries have packed up' across your forehead, so who's going to know you're different?

Women with premature menopause represented themselves as being caught in a dilemma between being old (menopausal) and being young. Young tended to be constructed as 'me', but being menopausal was construed as 'not-me', since this would mean taking on board being asexual, unfeminine, unproductive and of little value:

> I was still quite young. I'd thought of women my mother's age, of life ending or moving towards the end of your life, options closing down – now obviously I see it differently.
>
> It didn't concern me. It would happen at some point when I was older. Now I feel a lot different about it, thinking God, why me?

The challenge to identity was complicated by the fact that the menopause had arrived so unexpectedly, leaving the women feeling vulnerable and exposed. Several reacted proactively by, for example, changing their diet, not using caffeine, taking vitamins, exercising more, etc. The negative image of menopause was rarely completely accepted:

> All the photographs of grannies with greying hair – I couldn't identify with that. They talked about this stage of life when children are leaving home, and here I was, my child had just arrived.

Women described a variety of strategies used to deal with the impact of a premature menopause. One way was to take in what had happened in smaller, more manageable chunks:

> Dealing with it slowly and making small realisations, because it's too big a thing to deal with all at once.

Or to make a great effort to look on the bright side:

> You have to keep thinking positively all the time, if you start thinking negatively, you just drift down (tearfully).

Another was to highlight material advantages and freedoms:

> If I ever do feel a bit bad about it, which I do, I just remind myself about what's good about it. We can move where we like, don't have to worry about school or the expense, and can go on holiday two, three times a year.

Several hinted that premature menopause was experienced, either directly or indirectly, as a stigmatized state. Feelings of embarrassment or being devalued may be both a reflection of social attitudes and internalized shame:

> There's still a social stigma, it's still something people try to push under the carpet.

There was also evidence of indignant defiance at the perception of menopause as a social stigma:

> It's unbelievable – you'd think you've got AIDS or cancer or something, they're so frightened about it.

Generally a premature menopause was experienced as a private event, to be disclosed to a chosen few in selected circumstances. The need to maintain conventional self-presentation was repeatedly stressed:

> I want people to see me as I am. I don't want them to think it's like a huge part of me.

Whether or not the women discussed their menopause depended on situational context, possibly revealing their own ambivalence about how this reflected on themselves or themselves and their partner:

Very few people know. I just feel it's nothing to do with anybody else. If I can't
have children, well that's personal as far as I'm concerned. My partner's very
anti the idea of anybody knowing – not because he's embarrassed – but because
he thinks it's totally personal. And that, of course, affects how I talk about it.

However, most successful as a counterfoil to negative stereotypical
beliefs were attempts to bridge the gap through conversation with
others. The sense of personal and social isolation was exacerbated
where there was not at least one intimate and confiding relationship
to act as a protective buffer. This could be a partner, friend, someone
else who had experienced a premature menopause or a health
professional. There appeared to be a consensus that the psychological aspects of a premature menopause needed to be addressed swiftly
by health professionals – at, or close to, the time of diagnosis, possibly with periodic follow-ups to mitigate the accompanying
emotional pain and distress:

I really felt alone, battling along not knowing what was happening.

I don't know anybody else in my age group who this has happened to.

The majority felt that it would be useful to know others, either within
their own family or among their circle of friends who were in the
same menopausal 'boat':

It would have been helpful to have someone of the same age to talk to.

A supportive partner seemed to moderate the experience:

Basically, he's very kind, very patient and he makes me talk about it.

Although even when there seems to be support and sharing, communication can be difficult. A partner might not clearly understand the
significance of a premature menopause. For instance, it was only
after learning that she needed to let her partner know, through sharing her experience of premature menopause in a therapeutic group,
that one woman felt able to handle her feelings more satisfactorily
with her partner:

He didn't accept it, he didn't see it even as a painful event, or a loss. When I
spoke to him he said: 'I never realized that you want to, that you need to.'

The women in the present study expressed a heartfelt desire for peer support:

> It cheered me up when my GP said: 'I've got two other women on my books, one in the mid-twenties, one in her early thirties going through it too.'

> It's nice to know there's other people out there who have gone through, or are going through, the same thing – that you're not on your own. If you think you're on your own it makes it worse.

> If I'd known other people who had actually experienced it, it would have helped enormously.

However, there were also women wary of the idea:

> I'm self-contained anyway. Maybe other people who are feeling wobbly need to be able to off-load. I don't, I get things out of my system myself.

Counselling may help a woman to negotiate the healthcare system and enable her to ventilate feelings of anger and frustration without fear of burdening family and friends. Five of the women interviewed had found counselling helpful:

> I could say things I couldn't possibly say to my family – because it might upset them again and they'd been through enough. They don't want me hammering their heads against a wall again. So, it was an outlet.

> It probably made me aware of the things that I still do have, which is important to be aware of.

A sixth woman was planning to enter counselling some time in the future.

Overall, the experience of premature menopause can appear similar to that of mid-life menopause. Both are physiological processes or events that are varied, multidimensional and influenced by sociocultural context. A premature menopause, however, tends to be experienced as initially shocking and upsetting. For the majority of women a premature menopause implied major consequences in terms of reproductive capacity, concerns about ageing and future health, and their sense of identity as women. The women made use of health services and described both positive and negative views on the medical advice and treatment they had been offered. The need for information, good communication and sensitivity from health professionals was frequently mentioned, and welcomed when encountered. On the whole, premature menopause tended to be accompanied by a sense of loss – of health, youth, choice and the sense of being able to control the direction of their lives. However, emotional and material compensations could be found and unhelpful stereotypes were successfully challenged by at least some women. Emotional support and understanding from others, particularly friends, family and, for some, health professionals, was described as particularly important. However, there seemed to be a consensus that most helpful in dealing with premature menopause would be the opportunity to talk with other women facing similar issues and concerns.

Chapter 5
Behind the shut door: a psychoanalytic perspective

JOAN RAPHAEL-LEFF

'In my dream it's dark. I see nothing. I'm crying and there's this loud banging noise – then I realize it's me, pounding on the door of my parent's bedroom' says the woman on my couch. 'I feel frightened. Had a nightmare and want to come in their bed. But despite my yelling, my mother and father can't hear me. Maybe they're asleep, or having sex…Whatever. I feel left out, scared and angry – sobbing, calling, hammering on the shut door – but there is no reply'…

Dorothy and her partner have recently begun extensive fertility investigations with as yet inconclusive results. Increasingly, she feels they are living out a prolonged nightmare, emotionally ready for a baby but repeatedly failing to conceive. As her dream indicates, she feels 'left out, scared and angry', excluded from baby-making, and in her daily life suffers headaches, feels on the verge of tears all the time and finds it difficult to concentrate at work. Her sleep is disturbed by vivid dreams. She often wakes bathed in sweat, feeling anxious and experiencing palpitations. For almost a year now, as each cycle has drawn to its close, she and her partner have eagerly sought signs of conception, especially when her period was late, but sadly all the home pregnancy tests were negative. In recent months confusion has increased as her cycles have become irregular with spotting rather than periodic bleeding. She is unable to tell whether her symptoms are caused by tension at not conceiving and increasing unhappiness or are the cause of it. Her partner feels equally distressed and frustrated by their prolonged failure. Now he too is implicated as his sperm count when tested was found to be low.

Thirty-two-year-old Dorothy originally sought therapy shortly after her marriage, saying that she wanted to use twice-weekly therapy to explore a troubled relationship with her possessive mother as a prophylactic measure to avoid pitfalls with her own future baby. A year later, inexplicably excluded from fulfilling what had been taken for granted as a birthright, despairingly, she feels nothing in her life will ever be right again.

Dreams and the nightmare

Each of us, from infancy on, holds a tacit assumption that like our parents we have a natural capacity to make babies. We assume that within us the life-cycle trajectory of childhood, adolescence, adulthood awaits unfurling. And beyond that, parenthood and grandparenthood will follow if we so choose. Indeed, efficient contraception has fostered a widely held illusion of bodily control and self-determination. We believe we can decide whether to have a baby and designate the right time to conceive. An increasing number of individuals are choosing not to have children at all. Many other couples prefer to delay beginning a family or having another baby until they feel emotionally, professionally, economically and socially ready to do so. Some resort to abortion when an unplanned pregnancy occurs.

With discovery of fertility problems, suddenly the basic trust in one's control over generative potential is nullified. This is particularly poignant for a person who has decided the time has come to have a baby:

> 'You know' says Dorothy, after trying to conceive for almost a year, 'for a long time it wasn't that important to me to have a child. In fact earlier in my life I positively didn't want one, but now the desire is so intense it takes my breath away. The world is full of other people's babies. I also took it for granted I could just become pregnant. But why am I being denied? I'm not asking for something unreasonable – incredible yes, but not unreasonable...'

Dreams may reflect preoccupation with bodily symptoms before conscious awareness dawns. Even in those who have declined having children, the realization that something is wrong with their reproductive capacity provokes changes in familiar body image. No longer a taken-for-granted potential powerhouse, the body seems altered – ineffable, recalcitrant and mysteriously different. For people who wish to have a child, futile attempts to conceive add a painful dimension of frustration and irony at having used contraception for so long to avoid the very thing they now seek so avidly. To them the corporeal self seems to declare itself a separate entity – an unruly subversive traitor or ineffectual envelope to heartfelt desires.

Paradoxically, during fertility investigations the enigma is both heightened and dispelled with intensified self-scrutinizing and awareness of physiological processes. Bodily configurations are mechanized by postcoital tests and rudely invaded by endoscopic/sonographic observations which familiarize patients with internal aspects of their bodies hitherto unknown (such as the silent growth of individual follicles or thickness of womb lining).

Diagnosis

After investigations, eventually, the defining moment of diagnosis arrives:

> 'I can't bear it' cries Dorothy some days after being told she is becoming prematurely menopausal: 'I look around me and there's a whole world I can't get in to. No fairness! Why me? At first I felt like shouting at everyone: "If you can why can't I? I don't deserve another struggle!" It feels like an unjust punishment but there's no one to appeal to, and no one to blame...there's no rage any more, just helpless weeping – no point even in being angry with my body like I was before when I tried to coax it into working. I now know that whatever I do, I can't make it happen!'

Reeling with disillusionment, a person branded infertile may feel singled out – diminished by failure to fulfil the most fundamental prerequisite of the human race. Although for those who desire children, diagnosis of premature menopause need not mean lifelong childlessness, the reality is somewhat discouraging. New reproductive technology offers hope of child-bearing by means of ovum donation. However, there are few egg donors; the expensive treatments are beyond the reach of many, and its success rate is still only 30%. Adoption is another possibility particularly for young couples, but few newborn babies are available in countries where single motherhood is socially acceptable.

When a couple has been contemplating having a baby, in addition to her own grief, a young menopausal woman may also feel guilt-ridden at depriving her partner of a child. In her depression she might suggest separation to enable him to find a fertile mate, or even become preoccupied with suicide. He may indeed feel cheated of his

'birthright'. Their helplessness in the face of uncontrollable reproductive processes reactivates in their inner realities age-old painful
experiences of frustration, rejection and deprivation, infiltrating
their dreams and daily activities with a sense of futility. Tensions
often rise between partners as dissatisfaction and derision fester
below the surface or erupt in desperate attempts to regain equilib-
rium. Even where amicability is maintained it may be at a high cost
of denied expression. The couple's relationship may further deterio-
rate as discrepant emotions are revealed:

> 'I feel so isolated. Alone with this nightmare' cries Rachel, 'I call it that because I
> don't want it to be happening but can't make it stop. I still find it hard to believe
> we can't make a baby together but he doesn't seem all that bothered. Every
> morning I wake up again into the nightmare. In my dreams I am pregnant. In
> reality I am barren. It breaks my heart – but he says: "What's for breakfast?"'

Sexuality, sensuality and psychosexual representations are also
affected by the diagnosis:

> 'What's the point of having sex?' says Len, 'it's tame stuff. Can't lead any-
> where'...

Unable to bear the unbearable, would-be parents reel between
shock, denial, horror, rage, desperation and sadness. In a world now
divided starkly into haves and have-nots, fertile friends may be
resented. As confidence plummets, self-blame and/or accusations
proliferate, with each partner grabbing at wild explanations such as
illicit sexual encounters, previous terminations or undue postponement of child-bearing:

> 'I'll never forgive her if we've missed the boat', declares Simon. 'I was ready for a
> child years ago but she kept putting it off saying we couldn't afford it yet.'

One female anxiety experienced in childhood is a fantasy that internal reproductive organs have been damaged by the powerful archaic
mother in retaliation for her little girl's envious attacks on her
mother's fertility (Klein 1946). For some women, the situation of
infertility retriggers persecutory anxieties that resurface with a
vengeance, and premature menopause may seem both proof and
punishment for early destructive urges and forbidden desires. As
powerless to force conception as they were in childhood, a couple
may feel themselves becoming infantalized, once again excluded

from 'making babies' as they were from their mother and father's procreative relationship. Their rage may be focused on forbidding parents or the paternalistic doctors who are unconsciously targeted as free-floating oedipal anxieties find anchor in medical events. Others take their predicament in their stride. Why? I suggest that when unexpected infertility threatens the very epistomological centre of a person's world, what is at stake is generative identity.

Generative identity

'Generative identity' is a concept I proposed (Raphael-Leff 1995, 1997) as a fourth constituent of gender formation. The others are: core 'gender identity' (cf Money & Ehrhart 1972; Stoller 1985) – that is the mental representation of oneself as male or female; 'gender role' (cf Person & Ovesy 1983; Tyson & Tyson 1990) – relating to feminine or masculine psychosocial ideas of the self; and 'sexual partner orientation' (e.g. O'Connor & Ryan 1993), which focuses on articulation of hetero/homosexual desires. 'Generative identity', I suggest, constitutes a psychic construction of oneself as a potential progenitor.

I argue that generative identity means recognizing one's own reproductive capacities in the context of basic facts of life. It is consolidated between 18 and 36 months, when the child who previously imagined she or he could be 'everything' now has to face three basic restrictions – of sex (I am only female or male, not the other sex, neither or both), of generation (adults have babies, children cannot) and of generativity (females carry/suckle babies, males impregnate). For the toddler, these restrictions mean facing painful loss of omnipotence and relinquishing a belief in bisexual over-inclusiveness, resulting in acute feelings of jealousy towards adults and penis/womb envy of the other sex.

In other words, acquisition of generative identity entails mourning one's limitations: accepting being only one sex (rather than both and unlimited); pre-potent (rather than omnipotent) and only half of future procreative coupling (interdependent rather than autonomous). In two-parent families, it also means accepting that they have a sexual and reproductive union from which the child is excluded. Depending on emotional circumstances at this crucial time, the growing child may gradually accept the facts of life or may try mentally to rebel against these limitations by refusing their reality.

They may become inhibited by their pressure or engrossed in their compulsive re-enactment. I shall suggest that disturbances are more likely to occur when traumatic external events coincide in time with the critical period of demarcation of one's own generative potentialities.

Conversely, by achieving generative identity three momentous conceptual shifts become possible:

- a shift from being someone else's creature or creation to becoming a potential creator in one's own right
- freeing oneself from the biological determinism of sex by utilizing psychic cross-gender potentialities
- a shift from emphasis on physical procreativity of a baby to an abstract notion of creativity in general.

If these shifts take place, a person grows up with a sense of agency, feeling that irrespective of whether they are male or female, through identification with significant others they can encompass mental characteristics of both sexes without having to restrict themselves to being stereotypically 'feminine' or 'masculine'. And they can express their generativity in various non-reproductive ways rather than having to wait for a baby to fulfil it. Such a person may come to experience comprehensive gratification from creative expression of their wide-ranging potentialities, feeling no need to embark on parenthood.

When the sense of generative identity remains embedded in reproduction, having a child may come to seem the be-all and end-all of self-expression. To such a person, diagnosis of infertility can be particularly devastating. To a woman who has been living out her life in unconscious anticipation of child-bearing as the culmination of fulfilment, failure of procreativity threatens to generalize to all aspects of creativity, with loss of femininity as identity collapses into narrowly defined reproductive capacities. Despair sets in as the childhood promise of becoming creator of her own future child is broken.

Thus a woman who from early childhood has focused her female identity on pregnancy – taking for granted that when she grows up, like her mother's, her own egg will create a baby – may feel herself wiped out by premature menopause. Her basic trust is betrayed as ovulation ceases and abruptly ends the fertile years she had seen stretching ahead of her: eggs ripening in monthly succession, one of which would be chosen at the auspicious moment of fertilization when she felt absolutely ready to be a mother:

> 'I used to imagine my insides as this nice cosy place where the eggs all nestled waiting their turn' says Dorothy. 'Now it seems rotten in there. A dried-up wasteland and the nice round, full eggs are shrivelled, useless, empty duds...I'm a neuter! I can't even do what any bitch can. How can I feel feminine if I'm not even female anymore?'

Dorothy has a long emotional journey to restore her personal identity as a richly endowed and multifaceted woman who is not reliant only on egg production for a sense of her own creativity. Lifelong emotional difficulties with her competitive, judgemental and possessive mother have to be worked through to (re)gain a sense of herself as an autonomous insightful person as well as a potential mother. Further therapeutic work focuses on the relationship and ways of interacting that do not necessarily pivot on a child's genetic connection to her, but her capacity to give and receive love. Gradually, pleasure in her body's shape, sensuality and fitness replaces bitter disappointment at loss of the image of her laden figure swelling in pregnancy and ripening to give birth to her own baby as she herself had emerged from her mother's womb. Deciding not to pursue gamete donation, Dorothy and her husband are accepted on an adoption list.

Internal riches

Although in many cultures gender roles are clearly demarcated and stereotypically restricted, increasingly in the UK and the USA it is becoming acceptable for each of the sexes to demonstrate traits formerly reserved for the other. Females can now engage in assertive behaviour and pursuit of interests previously deemed 'unladylike', while males can be emotional, nurturing and sensitive in ways that were regarded as un-'masculine'. I suggest that for each individual, accessibility to the unique mix of internal richness is dependent on the degree to which their personal identity is freed from its strict male/female reproductive definition. This necessitates a tolerance of otherness, of difference, incongruity, contradictions and ambiguity within the self. Furthermore, I contend that it is never entirely stabilized and over our adult years cumulative experience is recurrently reworked at different times, with reinterpretation of various facets of one's own gendered identity, subjectivity, eroticism, sexual orientation and symbolic representations of generativity and fertility, feminine and masculine identifications and maternal/paternal capacities – all within an abiding sense of self.

This is the case with Dorothy (and her husband, too) as, during the course of her therapy, painfully relinquishing hope of a 'natural' child of their own, they each began to disentangle a firm sense of self from the gendered concepts inherent in physically producing a child. They could envisage themselves as potentially loving and gifted parents to a child not-of-their-making. Thoughtfully working through their own early experiences, they drew on their empathic understanding of each other to delineate the respective family constellations and unconscious dynamics that led to their fierce desire for a joint child. Distinguishing a subjective sense of a self from imposed gender definitions, genetics from nurturance, parenting capacities from reproductive ones, they could forego pregnancy without feeling failures or losing their respective senses of masculine or feminine identity while grieving the child they will never produce.

Ovum donation

Infertile couples find different solutions to their plight. Some adjust to infertility with relative ease, having resolved not to become parents. Others reluctantly accept involuntary childlessness, acknowledging the diminishing yet ever-present sorrow. Depending on the diversity of their internal worlds and the strength of sublimatory facets of generative identity, many eventually build on the richness of their lives and tap creative alternatives that do not involve parenthood. Some resolve to foster or adopt a child. Yet others find life together an intolerable reminder of their dashed hopes, and decide to separate, amicably or in bitterness. Other couples feel they must continue to make use of available medical treatment, pursuing with various degrees of hope or desperation, the conception that they feel will change their lives. When fertility treatment involves egg-donation, as it often does with premature menopause, complex conscious and unconscious factors come into play.

Sarah, a 37-year-old woman with no previous interest in 'deep' psychological understanding came to consult me some years into fertility treatment with donated eggs:

I have so much to be thankful for – my partner, friends, family, work. But my life has become consumed by this wish to have our…his…child. The more it doesn't happen, the more it becomes an issue. I became pregnant years ago when we first got together but had an abortion as we both were young and wanted to travel. We had such a great time together, just the two of us. We went all over the world, always together. Even when we came back home, for some years having a baby was a far-off thought. We enjoyed our life as a couple, didn't really want an intruder into our twosome. Then in our thirties it seemed a baby could be a happy bonus in our long relationship – an anticipated gift-to-come.

Now, after years of trying, there's a constant ache of something missing. Our house symbolizes it: in the years since we moved here I feel it acutely – this lovely big family house just waiting, empty. Time stands still. Most of the time, I do nothing. I'm scared I'll jinx it if I decorate a room for a baby. On the other hand, sometimes, I feel like rushing out to the shops and buying baby clothes. Crazy idea but it feels like the only way to break this suspended animation.

I suppose coming here to see you is another bit of magic. I'm menopausal but the doctors can't find a reason these eggs don't implant – so it must be in my mind. At times it feels as if I've lost interest in everything – my work, friends, my life – just despondent and waiting, always waiting… For a few months it was terrible, didn't feel like going out or seeing people … did nothing but cry. Felt it was unfair on my partner, tried to stop myself being so depressed, but the sadness is always there and sometimes I wonder if I feel if I'm miserable enough will this punishment be raised?

['punishment?' I repeat]

Sarah pauses thoughtfully:

I'm not sure why I said that. I guess when I was very young I felt punished when my mother left me on my own. I know she was busy with all the others and the housework as well, but I felt angry, left out – punished. I was the only one in the house who slept in a room by myself. They were all in pairs, my parents, my two older sisters and then when the little twins were born, they were always together, too. I used to creep down the hall and listen outside those shut bedroom doors – inside, each couple would be happy together, laughing or talking. And they all had babies – my sisters each looked after one twin; my mother and father had us; only I didn't have a baby. It's still true – they've all got children now. In fact, even my niece is pregnant. Only I'm still trying…

Funny, I remember when I was five and Dad told me Mum was expecting – it was like being kicked in the stomach. I still get that jolt when people tell me someone is pregnant – strange, goes right through me, as if madly jealous! Feels as if they're stealing MY baby from me! I try to be rational but everything seems so meaningful these days. When I hear that someone conceived – rather than feeling: 'Good! That means we've got a chance too!' it seems as though if they've got the baby we can't have it… [long thoughtful silence]

…I guess I still feel shut out…like that little girl standing folornly behind a shut bedroom door…

At her initial interview we had made an agreement for six sessions during which this hitherto unpsychologically minded woman began to trace connections with past suppressed feelings – permitting herself to open 'shut doors' in her mind. Gradually, as we explored less conscious aspects underpinning her hypersensitivity to feeling an outsider to a couple, we realized that there is yet another couple from which she now felt excluded – the joining of her husband's sperm and the donated egg. Not only was her partner 'betraying' the adult her with another woman to produce this baby, but the fertilized embryos in the lab Petri dish were also invested with powerful feelings from childhood when her mother betrayed her by joining forces with her father to create the twins. Finally, it seemed there was a fear of experiencing pregnancy, the symptoms of which she felt would remind her of her first unwanted pregnancy. All the cost and effort to procure pregnancy with a donor egg seemed a harsh rebuke to her partner and severe payment for the abortion in her teens, when they casually 'threw away' their potential baby. Two months after we ended our sessions she jubilantly phoned to tell me that she was pregnant.

When problematic issues remain unprocessed during an ensuing pregnancy, a donor-egg baby may continue to seem 'alien' to the mother or charged with intense ambivalence. In addition, there are practical and ethical dilemmas around ovum donation. According to the American Society for Reproductive Medicine, since the birth of the first baby by egg donation in 1984, an estimated 6000 women in the USA have given birth to babies conceived in this way. Some of these children are now of an age when the issue of disclosure is becoming a very real topic for debate (Stolberg 1998), with some mental health professionals and parents arguing that a child needs to know his or her origins. To them, withholding the information seems immoral, because family secrets can be devastating and/or because genetic histories are becoming increasingly important as scientists explore the hereditary aspects of disease. Others claim that the decision is deeply personal and to be made by each family after their own deliberations – which involve not only conscious considerations but unconscious forces too (see Chapter 9).

Life-cycle trajectory

If the psychoanalytic literature on menopause has been sparse, that on premature menopause is virtually non-existent. Classical psychoanalysis drew analogies between menopause and puberty as a time when, under the impact of hormonal changes, infantile conflicts around femininity, sexuality and maternal identification are revitalized and have to be reappraised before emotional tensions can be resolved (Deutsch 1924; Freud 1937; Benedek 1948). Recent revisions link the bleeding of menarche and its cessation in menopause to remobilized fantasies of both genital 'castration' and loss of female functions. In general, the 'climacteric' has been treated as a natural (albeit negatively charged) event in the life cycle rather than as a 'deficiency disease' (Notman 1995; Lax 1997). However, whereas previously menopause was seen to involve a process of 'desexualization' (Benedek 1950) it is now recognized that for some women, sexuality may be released and eroticism enhanced during and after the climacteric (Pines 1993). Similarly, in the past menopause was regarded as a 'narcissistic mortification' (Deutsch 1945) inevitably accompanied by depression. Today distinctions are drawn between transient depressive mood and clinical depression. It is accepted that only a minority of women experience the latter, mainly those with a history of depression (Panel report 1996). However, mid-life menopause is invariably associated with feelings about loss of the youthful self and bodily control during the processes of ageing (Lax 1982), sometimes exacerbated by the 'empty nest' syndrome of children leaving home. It is now generally accepted that the greater a woman's non-reproductive interests and activities, the less her self-esteem is affected by menopause. Indeed, for many women the 'change' of life may be a positive one, accompanied by 'expanded self-image' and increased wellbeing (Notman 1984), a potential spurt of maturational development as relief from pressures of sexuality and child-rearing offer opportunities for psychic growth (Pines 1993).

Clearly, the case of premature menopause differs. When the life-cycle trajectory is rudely interrupted, the suddenness of onset has a different effect to the long, gradual psychological preparation and physical decline of mid-life menopause. With menstrual pause, the cyclical rhythm by which a woman has marked time since puberty is disrupted. Unconsciously associated with age-old lunar mysteries and maternal identifications, to some, recurrent bleeding has represented proof of ongoing fruitfulness; to others, each period signified loss, of ovulation unfulfilled; or at times may have seemed a form of natural purification by 'blood-letting' or even a 'curse' inflicted on females alone. A study monitoring the content of dreams over different phases of the menstrual cycle (Benedek 1950) revealed the complexity of women's unconscious responsiveness to the ovulation–menstruation polarity. This relationship is often ambiguous – menses linked to relief or unconscious guilt over jettisoned hopeful internal growth, naturally excreted or wished away...ruby-red riddance of 'bad' accumulations that also provides repeated evidence of latent riches.

The emotional 'crisis' brought on by menopause may reflect exacerbation of a woman's unresolved ambivalence regarding her internal forces of creation and destruction. Be that as it may, if cessation of periods signifying the end of fertility can catch even an older woman by surprise, despite universality of occurrence and gradual forewarning, its effect on an unprepared younger woman may be very disturbing.

Fertility loss

With loss of fertility before reproduction, lineage ends. The infertile person falls off the generative trajectory of all the preceding generations, finding her or himself located at the end, rather than middle, of a chain of inheritance. While some people may have knowingly chosen this position by deciding not to have children, it is particularly shocking for a younger woman who has not yet fully contemplated the real choice of whether or not to have a baby:

> 'My whole future is smashed' sobs 19-year-old Sophie, recently diagnosed with a metabolic condition which has led to ovarian failure. 'My friends chat on about weddings, babies, clubs they've been to and boys they've met – but all those doors have been slammed in my face. I wish I was dead...No! I am dead – dead before I have even lived...' she wails inconsolably.

Not only does Sophie feel old before her time, but all her unrealized wishes, her nebulous hopes and dreams for 'one day' are suddenly rendered obsolete; her potential eggs evaporated long before their 'best by' date. She feels bewildered in a topsy-turvy world in which the older generation appears to have triumphed. How can anyone understand her plight – least of all her own mother who has been pregnant, has had a child and may still be fertile. Sophie feels isolated, baffled and betrayed; furious at no one and everyone, especially her mother who gave birth to a child with a genetic dysfunction. At 19, long before the mid-age watershed, Sophie confronts her extinction. It reverberates in her crie de coeur: 'I am dead' as mortality looms, no longer refracted through genetic continuity. On another level, seeking explanations, she wonders whether her bulimia has contributed to her condition and now sees her slim body as grotesque and mannequin-like – a celluloid doll with 'no insides'. She feels herself to be 'a female freak and fraud', no longer a budding, fertile woman but an 'empty shell', devoid of femininity, creativity, generativity. With the blow to her generative identity it will take many months of therapeutic self-exploration to work through her anxiety, rage, envy and profound sense of being cheated before she can accept that her value as a person is not diminished by her condition.

Compelling forces

While some women renounce child-bearing, others feel intensely that pregnancy is a quintessential female right and they cannot forego the experience come what may. Faced with the prospect of a hysterectomy, 28-year-old Maria is determined to have a child. So much of her feminine identity is invested in reproductive generativity that she feels unable to contemplate life without having been pregnant. She is a proud woman and much as she wants a child, is unwilling to enter a compromising heterosexual relationship for the sake of one. Wanting 'the best', she investigates the possibility of procuring a 'straw' of frozen semen from an American sperm bank advertising its sources as 'Nobel Prize candidates'. For some months her sessions in therapy are dominated by her trying to engage me in choice of the optimal 'gene father' for her baby ('The blue-eyed, blond engineer or the red-haired nuclear physicist?'). My interpretations that she seems to be wishing to replace her own absent father with an ideal fantasy one, fall on deaf ears. Gradually, through a dream of smothering a kitten, we begin to glimpse unconscious roots of her compulsion to have a child to replace the baby her mother lost to cot death when Maria was two years old. The baby was never mentioned again in the family and at times Maria thought she had imagined her existence. However, an aunt verifies her account and we begin to recognize how Maria's estrangement from her home reflects the sense of futility of her lifelong desire to compensate her bereaved, silent mother, driven by irrational guilt about having caused first her baby sister's death and then her father's desertion. As she accepts that her rivalry with her baby sister and childish fantasies of getting rid of her did not magically cause the infant's disappearance, the burden of her imagined transgression lifts and her compassion gives way to anger. She is flooded with rage at her depressed mother's emotional unavailability when, as a toddler, Maria too was grieving the loss of her little sister. Gradually her sense of rejection gives way to rage at her father's leaving them at such a difficult time. These internal changes enable Maria to make contact with her estranged mother and communicate with her in a way she felt unable to do while growing up.

Time is running out. Much remains unresolved in her therapy. However, faced with the prospect of a hysterectomy, Maria is nevertheless still resolved to have a child, both to continue the 'blood line' of her family and to heal her own childhood scars by giving a baby the happy childhood she feels she missed. The surgeon agrees that her operation can be postponed for one year and now that there is some flexibility, the loss of her uterus no longer seems another inflicted deprivation. Maria chooses to return to her country of origin and with her mother's help approaches a sperm bank of her own racial group, becomes pregnant with the first insemination and brings up her little girl in her mother's home.

This case and others like it raise the question of why faced with infertility, some women are able to resign themselves to mothering a genetically unrelated child or opt for childlessness (despite the availability of technological resources or possibility of adoption or fostering) while others cannot. In my view the answer hinges on developmental difficulties or traumatic events during the period of acquiring generative identity. In Maria's case, the sudden death of her baby sister during her toddlerhood confronted her with an irrevocable real disappearance that could not be rectified by desire for reparation and imaginary making good. Furthermore, her mother's prolonged emotional withdrawal and her father's leaving home seemed further to confirm for little Maria the destructive power of her own intense love/hate emotions, instigating a lifelong wish to create a real live baby to reverse the tragic events of her early childhood.

Power of the past

On the basis of intensive treatment of some 150 people seen between one and five times per week over the past 25 years in a psychoanalytic practice specializing in reproductive issues, I have found that the process of assuming generative agency is never fully completed. Reappraisals occur particularly during transitional phases in the life cycle – puberty, menstrual periods, pregnancy, childbirth and lactation, and menopause – when the distinction between female- and male-sexed bodies peaks unavoidably. Re-evaluations are also necessitated by crucial phenomena such as premature menopause or hysterectomy. As I have suggested, their effect will be intensified by the degree to which personal identity is invested in physical generativity (rather than sublimation).

When (as in the case of Maria) traumatic events have occurred during the critical period of a child's acquisition of generative identity (such as maternal miscarriage, obstetric complications, stillbirth, neonatal death, difficulties resulting in parental infertility treatment or childhood sexual abuse), generativity itself may seem fraught with dangers. Fears may result in phobic avoidance of child-bearing, by deadening of sexuality itself, or precipitous sterilization and/or other defensive obsessional measures reflecting a determination to control the uncontrollable destructive forces that seem inherent in procreativity. Other people may deal with the early trauma differently. Driven by a blind need to disprove their childish anxieties, they manically dice with danger. At times, this bravado over the internal generative conflict is played out in external reality – in promiscuity or recurrent acts of conception to prove fertility, followed by repeated abortions, which enact conflicts between life and death, creativity and destructiveness; or in driven sperm or egg donation realizing both powers of generosity and withholding. Clearly, to a person with this type of emotional history, miscarriage, subfertility or premature menopause will be particularly laden with psychic significance.

Clinical experience has led me to believe that when traumatic events coincide in time with the process of acquiring generative identity, unless the child is helped to process these events, she or he will resort to finding ways of concrete redramatization of the past event in present. I contend that the fact the trauma occurs in actuality rather than fantasy, propels a compulsion to re-enact it in reality. The child, and later the adolescent or adult, will go on attempting to secure unconscious expression of both the original trauma and its reparation through such externalized realization.

Enactment may take any of the forms mentioned above or may manifest bodily in psychosomatic ways, such as pseudocyesis ('pretend' pregnancy), psychogenic infertility or couvade symptoms in men who unconsciously mimic symptoms of pregnancy, miscarriage or labour. Other disturbances in generative identity range from rigid, gender-polarized self-representation of oneself as 'pure' feminine or masculine to concrete thinking and inhibited/deferred originality due to conflation of procreation and creativity; or grandiose disavowal of one or more of the facts of life, such as belief in 'immaculate' conception. These days enactment may be aided and abetted by use of new reproductive technologies which enable our wildest fantasies to be lived out in reality. In extreme cases, the compulsion to express the unprocessed trauma may culminate in such acts as impulsive baby-stealing, sexual or violent child abuse or even infanticide.

When premature menopause occurs in a woman who has not resolved generative traumata or internal conflicts from the past, these are likely to be retriggered and require therapeutic processing before she can adjust to the realistic implications of her current situation.

Conclusion

Dealing with unexpected infertility is always a major life event, whether it comes as the result of an ectopic pregnancy, surgical intervention or biochemical causes. It compels a re-evaluation of generative identity and forces a woman or couple to reappraise their sense of self, their expectations for the future and preconscious base for child-bearing decisions they have made and/or the ideal family they had imagined themselves creating. I have argued that some individuals who have chosen not to have children remain relatively unaffected by premature menopause. To others, and particularly those whose sense of generative identity is rooted in physical procreativity, the prospect of other options, be it creative sublimation, childlessness, adoption or fostering, is untenable as long as there is felt to be any hope of postmenopausal pregnancy. For many such women/couples, psychotherapeutic help during this critical period can be particularly beneficial. In addition to forestalling some of the relational difficulties that premature menopause may trigger between the partners, therapy consists of working through salient aspects of each person's psychohistory. By processing traumatic events and integrating split primary identifications, some people are enabled to transform a limited body-based system of generative identity into a sense of creative agency, which releases expression of multivariate facets of the self. In my clinical experience, this broader focus maximizes receptivity to medically assisted conception and the emotional issues involved. It also helps cushion against hopelessness when pregnancy is not a viable option by promoting the thoughtful capacity to unlock psychic 'doors' within the self rather than pounding on the physical one that has slammed shut.

Chapter 6
Difference and diversity

AGNES MARFO

The stories of many women experiencing a premature menopause are often unheard; particularly those of women from different ethnic backgrounds. It is easy to generalize about women's experiences and to make assumptions about peoples' beliefs and lifestyles on the basis of their religion or ethnic group. Moreover, women's experiences also vary along dimensions of age, sexuality and socioeconomic status.

There is a tendency to homogenize minority experience in a desire to find common ground (Aziz 1997). People in Britain 'have access to a wide range of...cultural practices that they can and do participate in' (Bakare-Yusuf 1997). One significant phenomenon apparent among the young is the extent to which black American and black Caribbean culture has permeated mainstream youth culture, not only of the majority community but also that of other ethnic communities. For example, the language of many young Asians in Southall and Birmingham is a cross between the local dialect, black American language and Caribbean patois (Luthra 1997). The group that individuals choose to identify with is likely to be

> ...in most cases [a case of] tactful accommodation particularly in the case of the young, leading to the notion of being culturally a Hindu or a Sikh, i.e. believing and belonging to the majority culture to a deliberate extent depending upon the situation (Luthra 1997)

I was interested in exploring how cultural perceptions and expectations surrounding issues of fertility, motherhood and women's roles might influence women's experiences of premature menopause. I interviewed two women, Nadia and Justine, who talked about their experiences of premature menopause within the context of their respective cultures (see Table 6.1). The other interviews, which were carried out with men and women (Table 6.2), illustrate the ways in which cultural values, attitudes and beliefs can influence a woman's experience of premature menopause. The views articulated in this chapter are not intended to be representative of any specific culture. Rather, they will reflect the range and diversity of beliefs and opinions regarding this subject within different ethnic communities.

Table 6.1: Details of the women diagnosed with premature menopause

Name	Age	Age when diagnosed	Marital status	Ethnicity	Religion	Country of birth	No. of children
Nadia	30	27	Married	Indian	Catholic	India	0
Justine	31	15	Single	Black British	Christian	England	0

Table 6.2: Men and women interviewed about their cultural beliefs and practices

Name	Age	Ethnicity	Religion	Country of birth
Vrinda	26	British Mauritius/Other	Telegu (sect of Hindu religion)	England
Sue	45	Asian	Sikh	India
Alka	32	Indian	Hinduism	England
Mohammed	34	Asian	Muslim	Uganda, East Africa
Ola	34	Black British (of Nigerian descent)	Muslim	England
Kwame	40	Ghanaian	Deist (believes in God not in a divinely revealed religion)	Ghana, West Africa

Vrinda, is 26; her family are from Mauritius but she was born in England. She felt that she had integrated well into mainstream British society while retaining her own cultural identity and traditions:

I usually call myself other or British Mauritius. I'm Asian-looking so refer to myself as Asian, but if people asked me what continent I come from I'd say Africa...I'm not like normal Asian girls. I smoke, I do everything against the norm. I'm not subdued. I'll wear long skirts, short skirts, traditional costumes as well as normal...I'm Telegu, which is a sect of the Hindu religion and I do like to (observe) religious practices like prayers and religious ceremonies and speak my own language – Creole.

Invariably, minority communities will lose traditional beliefs and values in the process of assimilation into the dominant culture. Sue, aged 45 is a Sikh, born in India. She has witnessed the transformation of her culture over the years with each generation:

For Sikhs, things have changed so much. We want to be Westernized, so we've changed so much. We have to change with the children otherwise we lose them.

The younger generation are constantly pushing boundaries and testing social acceptability. Sue, recalls how, many years ago, a family member was frowned upon by marrying outside her caste. Her 'transgression' changed family attitudes over the years. When Sue's daughter

was going out with another religion boy – he was a Sikh...but different...there are different categories

Sue's family were more tolerant. However, Sue worries that her girls may go:

...one step further than I'd like...In my time my marriage was arranged. Some families still have arranged marriages. There is still a stigma about people going out together. When my older daughter wanted to go out with this guy – it was restricted. We had to know the person...His family were invited round. They can't just make up their minds.

Despite having to accommodate and compromise certain cultural traditions, there is one that Sue is anxious for both her girls to observe:

Marriage is extremely important for Sikh girls. We like our girls to get married early. Not 18 or 19, but in their twenties because they're our responsibility while they're at home, financially and in all other aspects. We don't let them live away from home.

Some ethnic minorities appear to retain a high degree of separate identity and lifestyle from the majority culture and do not become fully integrated within it. Certain groups of Asian origin tend to fit this pattern. Thus, a large number of British Bangladeshis – notably in the Tower Hamlets area of London – do not speak much English and participate relatively little in life outside their own families and ethnic community (O'Donnell 1991).

The experience of a premature menopause can be particularly isolating for women who come from minority ethnic backgrounds. Statistically, they are in a minority of a minority and this naturally reduces the number with any specific experience to share. This can heighten feelings of difference and result in women feeling that they do not belong to any identifiable group.

This was evident during the interviews that I conducted with Nadia, an Indian woman aged 30, and Justine, who is black British, aged 31. Both were interviewed on two separate occasions for about two hours. Interviews were partly structured. I asked some questions focusing on their reactions to their initial diagnosis, reactions from family and friends and long-term concerns. However, these were mere guidelines used to generate conversations on areas of their lives that might have been affected by the onset of a premature menopause. The women were encouraged to steer the conversation by talking about issues that were important to them. Although I was eager to examine how cultural factors may have affected their individual experiences, I left it to the participants to determine the extent of its significance in their experience, if at all. The results are two very divergent stories.

Cultural comparisons were important to the participants in these case studies. They saw themselves primarily as Asian and black women diagnosed with a premature menopause. Both shared distress about fertility, feeling estranged from fertile women. Justine said:

> Sometimes being amongst women who have children makes me feel uncomfortable. It reinforces my feelings of inadequacy.

They described feelings of alienation from indigenous white women experiencing the same condition because they felt that white women were viewed more sympathetically. Nadia remarked:

> I think their culture is just so much more open and they can talk about these things.

Women within their own cultures were viewed at times as being less understanding and more judgemental. Nadia feared being the subject of community gossip:

> I find it easier to talk to people from other cultures. I honestly don't know why. I think mainly because I don't want them talking about me. I just feel they'll be saying, 'Oh poor girl'.

For some women, the experience of a premature menopause does not transcend cultural barriers. Nadia is Indian. She grew up in Botswana but now lives in Britain. She is unable to identify with the experiences of white women as she feels her concerns are culturally specific:

> It's always different for women of colour.

Nadia has rejected counselling as a suitable option for her, feeling that no one can help and that she has to deal with problems in the context of her culture:

> Nobody's said anything I didn't already know. I think it's something I have to deal with and work out for myself. I know what the problem is and I've got to deal with it. Just think I've got to do it my own way.

Nadia is from a culture that is fundamentally family orientated:

> Our culture revolves around family.

She relishes the opportunity to be a part of that tradition. As far as she is concerned, the worst aspect about having an early menopause is being infertile:

> All I ever wanted out of life was to be married, be a wife and have children. I never wanted to be rich or have a big job.

Other lifestyle choices adopted by many women in Britain, being single, 'married and childless', 'married and child-free', are not acceptable options for women within Nadia's community:

> Having children, it's like a woman's lot in our culture. Your whole life is to get married, be a good wife and then have children.

When women's roles are so narrowly defined, the pressure placed on them to conform is intense. Nadia is constantly reminded of her 'duty' as a newlywed.

From the day I got married, 'When are you having a child?'

Her role expectations are continually reinforced by other women. Nadia recounts a poignant moment while on holiday in India:

> When I went back to India I can remember going to church with my mum. An old women just came up to me and stabbed me in the stomach...You see, the only reason married women go back to their mother is if they're pregnant. Women go to their parents when they're seven months pregnant and go back home when the child is three months old. This old woman asked me 'So when are you planning to start a family? When are you expecting?'

Nadia is adamant that she will not return to India as she fears the constant probing into her private affairs:

> I don't even want to go back, not even for a holiday. My parents think it's stupid, but I just feel they'll keep asking me, make it really hard. You can't tell Indian people to mind their own business basically. They just want to know about us. It's a cultural thing.

The impact of infertility associated with a premature menopause can be exacerbated by cultural expectations and established roles for women. Infertile couples confront the lack of an appropriate 'cultural script' (Kirk 1984) for their childless situation. The cultural script prescribes biological parenthood for the legally married within a 'cultural timetable' (Erickson 1966). Deprivation, dissonance and culture shock result when the infertile recognize the discrepancy between the cultural script they have learned and the personal reality of involuntary childlessness they are forced to confront. Although the infertile (in contrast to the voluntary childless) conform to motivational norms by wanting children, they violate behavioural norms by not having them. The infertile are, therefore, deemed culturally deviant (Veevers 1972).

Each community places a different value on fertility, as does each individual. Alka, aged 32, is a Hindu Punjabi. She understands the pressure placed on women in India to conceive within the first year of marriage:

> If after one year you've not had children, people will question, 'Are you barren?' Women are supposed to bear children and there is a stigma attached if you can't have children. [Assisted reproduction] such as artificial insemination is frowned upon.

However, she believes that the perceptions of fertility problems among Asians in Britain are different:

> I'm not sure it's quite the same here...It all depends on where you're living in England. If you're in London, it's much easier than if you're living in the Midlands. It has to do with how people form their ideas and stereotypes. London is more cosmopolitan and there is a range of views. It also depends on your peer group and the kind of organizations you belong to. People here view things differently.

Sue explains that in her community:

> There is no stigma whatsoever. Infertility is recognized. I think in the past there was a stigma, many years ago in my mum's time, not anymore. Families are so important to us because we believe family is unity. When you're in trouble people will rally round. Someone's only got to be ill and people just rally round. If you can't have children you just go for help like anybody in this country would, but there's no pressure.

Nadia, who was diagnosed with a premature menopause at the age of 27, has always received support from her husband and immediate family members:

> I come from a very strong close-knit family. They've been very supportive. You'll never hear about an infertile man in our community. It's always the woman's fault. I did say to my husband, 'What if I tell them it was your problem and not mine?' He says 'If that's what you want, if you think the pressure's going to be less on you, tell them.' I was so amazed.

Faith is a constant source of strength for her:

> I suppose (what has been) most helpful has been my mum and prayer and faith. I've got a grand-aunt who's a nun and the whole convent keep saying prayers. She's 92 years old and she can't see now and she'll dictate letters to a young nun to write to me and say we're praying for you, just little things like that which keep me going.

Perceptions of fertility also differ among men across caste, religion and nationality in the Asian subcontinent. Aware of the options available to Muslim men married to infertile women, Nadia, one day presented her husband with a choice:

> If I was Muslim I'd worry because men are allowed to have four wives. I did offer to divorce my husband. I understand that most men would like to see children of their own. I told him 'You're very welcome to get married again to whoever you like.' He told me, 'Don't be stupid. Divorce is not an option.'

Mohammed is a Muslim. He does not have children but echoes Nadia's husband's sentiments:

> It certainly wouldn't bother me if my partner or wife couldn't have kids. There are lots of kids who need a home and a family. It's just a case of you loving the kids and the kids loving you, of them becoming yours and you becoming their father.

He argues that how individuals form their concept of role and place in society will influence their veiws on this subject:

> If a person has stronger religious ties they wouldn't be bothered by infertility, if they have stronger cultural ties they will...On the Indian subcontinent it would bother them more because it's an issue to do with culture rather than religion.

Mohammed regards the influence of culture on an individual as the 'weaker part of the community' and religion 'as a guide to life':

> My cultural element has been dissolved...I'm two generations away from the Indian subcontinent and then when I came to England, I was even more removed. I don't see my identity as being linked to roots because I have very few roots...my roots were in Africa, but looking at me you wouldn't believe that. All my friends were African, dark-skinned, I had an African nanny...'

Like so many immigrants and minorities trying to negotiate different, often conflicting cultures, Mohammed, has forged his own identity:

> I don't know if my perspective on things is conditioning and living in England or living in London, but I regard myself as British Muslim. I live by the rules of my faith.

Mohammed, has no qualms about adoption because his religion 'allows adoption freely'.

Justine was 15 when she was diagnosed with primary amenorrhoea. Her parents are from West Africa. She was born in England and refers to herself as black British. She is now 31 years old and has:

> ...finally come to terms with my medical condition as a result of yearly follow-up sessions with my gynaecologist and...counselling.

In the past, the crux of Justine's problem lay in her inability to reconcile her identity as both a female and a woman. She identified easily with other females since her 'chromosome constitution' (de Beauvoir 1987) had made her one. Although she described having the female characteristics of many other women:

> I have the same sexual characteristics as other women...breasts, a uterus, ovaries

she still saw her identity as separate, feeling that she somehow lacked the credentials to be a woman:

> Until recently I didn't consider myself to be a real woman...I felt deficient.

In her attempt to define 'woman', de Beauvoir (1987) said that:

> It would appear, then, that every female human being is not necessarily a woman; to be so considered she must share in that mysterious and threatened reality known as femininity.

Justine remarks:

> Before I started to develop breasts, I often felt uncomfortable and awkward about my own body image. I would rarely wear dresses as I had no breasts and felt that dresses were so unflattering. I had no curves and in jeans I looked like a boy...I remember an incident in my early teens. I was out shopping with a friend. It was a chilly day, my hat flew off and I lost it to the wind. I remember a woman shouting, 'Look! That boy's lost his hat!'

In her twenties, Justine tried to reinforce her femininity so that there could be no ambiguity about her identity:

> I didn't do it in an overpowering way...just a little make-up, a bit of jewellery. I suppose I was conforming to stereotypical ideals but when you don't feel like a woman or feel particularly feminine you begin to think that everybody else has that impression of you too. I really didn't want to go back to those days when I felt like a rare breed...flat-chested, no periods...when I was different...I just wanted to blend in.

Her attempts did not altogether make her feel like a woman, but she says:

> I may have been accepted as a woman in the eyes of others.

Those feelings she attributes to the absence of her 'first rite of passage' (Stepanich 1992), which she considers vital in constructing a healthy adult female identity. Perhaps no rite of passage is more significant to a young girl than menarche, since this marks the beginning of several transformative phases in the life of a young girl –

discovering a new self-identity, an awareness of sexuality, embarking on personal relationships.

> ...The first bleeding [the] initiation into the honor of womanhood [is] an extremely significant part of a young woman's experience, because what is experienced at this time will permanently be imprinted on our psyche. It is this imprint that will influence how we feel about our menses, our sexuality, and inevitably the stance we take toward our womanhood.
>
> (Stepanich 1992)

Moreover, how girls or women perceive and respond to menstruation and menstrual change derives very largely from their reference groups and the culture in which those groups are embedded. Some girls and women are socialized to accept menstruation as their biological fate rather than as an affirmation of [their] womanhood. Menstruation is seen by some women as a necessary evil so a woman can have a baby and as a fact of life, 'I'm indifferent: I know I've got to have them, so I put up with them' (Scambler & Scambler 1993).

In some societies menstruation is eagerly anticipated. In order to explore views about menstruation and menarche, I interviewed Dr Ocansey, who has worked in many hospitals in Ghana, West Africa, as a general doctor (general practitioner). He first came into contact with women experiencing a premature menopause at the Komfo-Anokye hospital in Ghana, where he trained. He explains the importance attached to menstruation in many African societies:

> In some parts of Africa, schistosomiasis (a parasitic disease which causes bloody urine) is very prevalent. Most of the boys normally play in the streams and they get bilharzia (an older term for schistosomiasis) and they urinate blood. That's one common sign of bilharzia and in some cultures it's very normal for all boys to urinate blood because they feel that it's a form of menstruating. So if you are a boy and you don't even have blood in your urine, they feel it's abnormal. That's the mentality that some people have and the same thing happens with women.

Late maturation can cause anxiety among girls who 'may feel immature and childlike...' (Petrie 1990). Dr Ocansey describes how the status of the young girl is enhanced in Ghanaian communities by the onset of menarche:

> In Ghana...a female or a girl is accepted as a woman when she starts menstruating. Let's say you are living in a village or within a compound house, a community...and you're of age but you haven't started menstruating. Nobody regards you as a woman, so if people younger than you start menstruating before you do, you'll be subject to ridicule. People will ridicule you, nobody will regard you, no

man will even be interested in you because if you don't menstruate you are just a girl, you're not yet a woman.

Among the Aowin people of southwest Ghana, 'the woman's initiation rite, the menzeua "is performed" after a girl has begun to menstruate and marks the commencement of her sexual life...By the performance of this rite, the Aowin people define their expectations of a woman's fertility'(Ebin 1982).

Pressure to conform to gender role behaviours comes from both men and women within a culture. Every person is socialized with certain role expectations. These are gender-based and reinforced from the earliest age by words and acts of the parental generation and by approval or disapproval of the child's behaviour. There is also some evidence suggesting that girls may experience difficulty in asserting their individuality. For example, Orbach (1998b) commented on recent national responses of little girls to Geri Halliwell aka Ginger Spice, and her split from her 'Spice mates'. 'It's stupid for Geri to fight and they should just get back together' said one girl. According to Orbach, what this indicates is that:

> When it comes down to it, young girls don't find the spectre of differentiation much easier than their mothers do...The need to confirm identity through sameness runs deep...

Peer pressure and a desire to belong and identify with other groups of teenagers are factors that encourage uniformity.

Throughout her teenage years, the young girl gains a deeper insight into her sexual identity and 'what membership of that group implies' (Yorburg 1974). Justine describes how her lack of participation in the exclusive adolescent world led to feelings of displacement as a youngster:

> I didn't feel that I belonged anywhere. I didn't fit in with any particular group. I couldn't talk about periods because I didn't have them...boyfriends because I didn't have one...I didn't get to wear a bra until I was 19...People made odd comments about my lack of development, but they didn't exclude me...I just felt inferior to other girls...I had all these expectations. I kept waiting for my period, then I'd develop breasts, then I'd look more attractive to boys...I might get a boyfriend and be the same as other girls...I felt that those were the things that were supposed to be happening to me.

Pre-pubescent girls are able to lead autonomous lives. This is the time in life when it is quite permissible for girls to be 'tomboys'. But as they move towards and into adolescence, they feel and respond to pressures that point them in a more 'feminine' direction. They internalize much of their role without even being aware of it. Increasingly, age and experience have given them an idea of how life is organized and they begin to structure their present and future perceptions accordingly. The switch from masculine preferences to feminine ones can be rationalized through shared involvement in the social trappings of femininity and through acknowledging the more enjoyable aspects of being female. This has already started happening for many children before they reach their teens, aided by earlier puberty and easy access to information about sexuality and womanhood (Sharpe 1994).

As a late developer, Justine equated her absence of periods with deficiency:

> I felt I wasn't functioning properly.

Negative associations are evident in medical terminology:

> Menopause is seen as a failure or breakdown of central control: ovaries become 'unresponsive'; the hypothalamus begins to give 'inappropriate orders'. When fertilization fails to occur, the endometrium is shed, and a new cycle starts. This is why it used to be taught that 'menstruation is the uterus crying for lack of a baby'...conceptualizing menopause as a kind of failure of the authority structure in the body contributes to our negative view of it...
>
> (Martin 1990)

In her late teens Justine:

> worried about whether or not a man would be interested in me if I told him I couldn't have children...I don't know if I really wanted children. I just felt redundant because I was unable to have them.

Many of Justine's contemporaries expected to have children at some stage in their lives. She often told friends that she expressed no interest in having children of her own much to their surprise – 'What...so you want to grow old on your own?' or 'Why? After you there'll be no one.'

For young women growing up in the 1990s, choices relating to the issue of motherhood may appear less problematic. It no longer seems 'necessary to defend women's right not to have children' (Mitchell & Oakley 1986). For Justine the issue of infertility needs to be understood in the context of a culture that places a great deal of emphasis on motherhood:

> In West Africa, in order to become a socially recognized adult, even in some cases to have proper mortuary rites performed, a woman or man must first become a parent, and tremendous pressures are exerted on these deviants who postpone the event beyond the age regarded as normal. Marriage is meant for child-bearing...Infertility results in acute anxiety, and a search for ritual and medical assistance...Parenthood provides the pivotal social role for individuals.
>
> (Oppong 1987)

Dr Ocansey, describes infertility as a:

> very dreadful social condition. People [in Ghana] will accept early menopause but the infertile woman is sometimes an outcast. Nobody will sympathize with her.

This is because infertility is commonly associated with pelvic infection attributed to promiscuous behaviour. It creates much concern and anxiety among family members according to Dr Ocansey:

> If a woman gets married and for a year she doesn't produce a pregnancy, society is worried. Who is society? Society is the man's family. The man's family is worried because they don't see why their son should get married to a woman who cannot achieve a pregnancy to continue their lineage. The woman's family will be worried because they know that their daughter has a problem and that is going to be the beginning of ridicule. Everybody's going to start pointing accusing fingers at them. The woman's mother is going to have a big headache on her head because they're going to tell her that she didn't bring up her child well... because the child was so promiscuous that's why she might have had so many abortions and because of that she's infertile...Every time people marry, people are always waiting. Twelve months and they want to see something...The woman will be going to become pregnant at all costs. She must prove her fertility and hence her fidelity before she got married.

Similar attitudes are held by Nigerian women:

> a barren woman was seen as a person apart, different from the rest, a mere onlooker...There is an assumption that fertility is normal and a barren woman 'deviates' or 'turns' towards barrenness. Misuse of the body, including promiscuity and abortion, are often thought to be the major cause of infertility. Life is not viewed as worthwhile without children.
>
> (Ladipo 1987)

It is difficult for many women to ignore the demands of community expectation. Ola is 34. She was born in England but has lived in southern Nigeria in the state of South Ogun for five years. Although she already has children, there is still pressure from family members to achieve another pregnancy, preferably two pregnancies:

> Everyone's telling me that I have to have one more at least, but I can't afford to have another one...A woman has to have kids...nothing like I don't want to have kids ...it's like a stamp on a woman if she doesn't...Back home there's pressure everywhere you go...here a woman is safer, she can hide behind her career.

Some African men seek confirmation of a woman's fertility and view it as a necessary prerequisite to marriage. Kwame, who is 40, was born in Hohoe, the Volta Region of South Ghana. He has lived in England for over 20 years:

> I wouldn't like to be married to a woman who couldn't have children. I would like to know that she could have children before we got married...If she couldn't have a child I'd ask her if she wouldn't mind if I had a child with somebody else. If she did mind, I'd leave her...If the fault was mine, it wouldn't bother me if she left me to have a child with another man.

He explains the 'overwhelming burden placed on families to produce children' as part of a continuation of a tradition that emerged initially from economic necessity:

> I think it goes back to the days when children used to help on the farms and they were seen as an asset and a property rather than a loving addition to the family.

Ladipo (1987) cites economic considerations as the principle reason behind procreation in modern-day Nigeria:

> The most frequently mentioned advantage of having children was security: financial security for old age and assurance of conjugal status in the husband's house. These two advantages (mentioned by 16 women) were often seen as inter-meshed in that the older the woman, the greater the probability of her husband dying and leaving her without a home support. A child ensures her right to live in the father's house and should also provide some financial support. Furthermore, a childless woman has no access to any inheritance from her husband but a mother will receive his wealth indirectly through her children.

The social consequences of involuntary childlessness can appear harsh. The individuals have not chosen their fate, yet are chastised by society for failing to adopt their assigned roles. In some instances, people may feel socially excluded:

It becomes evident that, in relation to the family, the childless will take on a secondary role, on the periphery...peripherality is the experience of those who stand on the edge of the society they wish to join: Peripherality leaves them with an absence of role within the family; a sense of not belonging, and being of little importance in the family; a need to search for alternatives that are not typical for their generation; and a struggle to discover what their life can mean if they are to have no part in rearing a new generation.

(Houghton & Houghton 1984)

Although the concept of 'peripherality' is less relevant to Justine's life, she does empathize with those individuals experiencing that kind of isolation. Many of Justine's friends have recently married or settled down with long-term partners and are considering or have started families. The distancing between herself and very close friends came without warning:

One minute we were speaking continuously on the phone and meeting up frequently...then after marriage and children they seemed to disappear. I took it very personally at first. It upset me a lot. I felt as though they had no need for me...Now I accept that their lives have moved on in a different direction to mine.

Justine's infertile status and how this may impact on future relationships used to be a major concern:

I made all sorts of assumptions that men would reject me...that they would reject me because I can't have kids...I'm sexually inexperienced...I've stopped worrying now. My gynaecologist and counsellor told me that lots of men would have relationships with women who can't have children. I only really began to believe that when I confided in men. There was no particular reason why I chose to tell some men and not others...Sometimes I felt obliged to. When they'd ask me about past relationships I'd clam up. I've never had a boyfriend and I'd justify why not. I'd tell them that my fear of rejection had stopped me from pursuing relationships. It was totally inappropriate but I thought that if I didn't say anything, they'd think I was weird.

The reactions of black men particularly surprised her:

I was always led to believe that black men might be put off pursuing a serious relationship with a woman if she couldn't have kids...In my experience this hasn't been the case. I've only ever told three men and all have been black. Two were Nigerian, one had been born over there...they were all very understanding. The other guy a West Indian couldn't understand why 'I was making such a big deal...Men don't worry about these things nowadays'.

From Justine's experience it may be that contemporary views among black men on the subject of infertility are varied and possibly changing, and illustrates why assumptions should not be made about people's views on the basis of their race or culture. Perhaps these views were widespread and shared by many men who may not necessarily have had the opportunity to articulate them. Often within minority communities one view is upheld as the authoritative voice of the community and considered representative. What is apparent is that the economic constraints that bound many African women to motherhood in the past are not always applicable in the lives of many African women living in Britain today. Education and social and economic mobility are presenting those privileged individuals with more options. Men and women are starting to question their traditional role expectations and its relevance in their lives. New identities are being constructed and alternative life courses pursued.

Justine's view of herself has changed dramatically over the past year. She says with a final sigh of relief:

> I've got rid of all that baggage...all those negative feelings about myself. They were just holding me back. I'm looking forward to the future with optimism. I've felt like this for nearly a year now so I hope that this is really the final turning point. I don't want to focus on my infertility. When I meet the right man I'll tell him and we'll move on...I feel better about my own self-identity now. I just see myself as a woman with a medical condition. I could have been diagnosed with any other condition. Mine just happens to be primary amenorrhoea. I've been lucky. I've had access to good and continuous medical assistance over the years, which I needed. I've never had any kind of interference from my family and extended family members. My parents leave me to get on with my life. They've never made my infertility an issue. It was mentioned in the early stages of my diagnosis when they were very upset...they've both told me how devastated they felt at times. If I want to talk to them about it I will. My mum says that if I want to adopt, then I should...I wouldn't go for egg donation personally. There are too many ethical considerations to think about. If I had the financial resources I would adopt. Money would be an important consideration because I would want to devote my time to bringing up a child...My dad says I shouldn't let this matter disrupt my life. I can still get married – which is something I think I really would like at some stage in the future – and lead a happy life without children.
>
> I've started to build an active social life which I think has contributed towards my healing process. I haven't forgotten my old friends who have settled down but I now accept that I may only get to see them three or four times a year. That's OK...and when we meet up I'm sure we'll have a great time – as I recently did with one friend – as there's loads to catch up on. In my twenties I spent too much time dwelling on how other people might react...it did nothing but hold me back and make me depressed. I've made a new life for myself. I've got hobbies that I actively pursue, I try and do activities where I meet people...a job that I enjoy, personal ambitions that I'm setting out to achieve. I've set out to cultivate this life and am creating my own happiness in the process. I think

though that once you accept the cards that have been dealt you in life...it liber-
ates you.

Justine's inability 'to live up to' her 'prescribed script' was, she main-
tains, responsible for many of her negative experiences as a girl and
woman.

> With the continued spread of individualism, humanism, and equalitarianism in
> modern societies... The terms masculinity and femininity will disappear from
> modern languages because they will no longer reflect standards that guide
> thought, emotion, and behavior. The primary source for such standards will be
> the individual and his or her temperament and abilities – these factors alone will
> determine the roles and the identities of human beings, regardless of gender.

(Yorburg 1974)

The stories in this chapter illustrate how cultural expectations can
influence women's experiences of premature menopause. They also
highlight the importance for health professionals to acknowledge
differences among individuals from ethnic communities. The views
expressed can be used to challenge preconceived ideas about women
from minority cultural backgrounds and their experiences of premature menopause. Every woman's experience of menopause is unique
and requires an individual approach and strategy of care management. It is therefore incumbent on health professionals not to make
assumptions about women's experiences on the basis of their ethnicity or religion but instead to be open to difference and diversity in
relation to a premature menopause in the context of sociocultural
beliefs and practices.

Part 3
Treatment approaches

Chapter 7
Management of premature menopause in general practice

JEAN COOPE

> I am 27 years old and my periods stopped two years ago. The GP in my previous practice said that it wasn't important if I didn't want to get pregnant. Do you think I should do something about it?

This actual question from a patient's history is one type of presentation of premature menopause to the general practitioner. A young woman below 40 years of age, with a previously regular cycle, experiences over six months of amenorrhoea (no periods). A pregnancy test is negative. Others may cite extremely irregular periods and in these cases, amenorrhoea for over a year is regarded as the criterion for investigation for premature menopause. Women whose ovaries are irradiated or removed surgically as part of a planned operation for the treatment of endometriosis, ovarian malignancy or benign cysts will also experience premature menopause.

A much more traumatic situation occurs when oophorectomy is carried out without proper discussion with the woman concerned, who may be devastated after a hysterectomy to find that in addition to losing her uterus she has also been deprived of her ovaries. The following correspondence between a gynaecologist and GP was quoted as justification for this approach:

> While I was in there I decided it was better to take it all away, rather than have to go back in later if she develops ovarian cancer.
>
> (Menage 1994)

Such prophylactic oophorectomy is common. Unfortunately it may not always be adequately discussed before or after the operation and in such circumstances is likely to cause women profound emotional turmoil.

Investigation for premature menopause

Women with premature menopause frequently report vasomotor symptoms such as hot flushes, night sweats and secondary insomnia, and fatigue and emotional distress. Also, a reduction in libido (sexual drive) can follow loss of ovarian androgens. These symptoms can be more acute in young women than in women with an on-time menopause. All these different situations require a range of diagnostic skills and management. In particular the practitioner needs to be aware of the emotional impact on the person experiencing a very early menopause.

Conditions to consider before making a diagnosis of premature menopause include:

- pregnancy
- prolactinoma
- medication, e.g. after combined oral contraceptive (COC) pill, during progestogen contraception, levonorgestrel intra-uterine device (IUD) or injections; chemotherapy for malignancy; treatments for endometriosis such as danazol and Gn Rh analogues
- patient is in the postpartum phase and/or breast-feeding
- pituitary and hypothalamic insufficiency due to anorexia nervosa and excessive weight loss, marathon running, severe psychological distress
- endocrine disease, e.g. abnormal thyroid function
- polycystic ovary syndrome
- premature ovarian failure (POF), often associated with chromosomal abnormalities.

A medical history should include date of last menstrual period, whether menses were previously regular and whether the woman is taking medication or had irradiation or chemotherapy. The family history may include a history of premature menopause.

Physical examination would include measurment of height and weight, inspection for abnormal hair distribution, examination of breasts and, if possible, vaginal examination to exclude pelvic mass.

The following tests should be considered:

- pregnancy test
- serum prolactin should be measured and, because stress increases prolactin (a hormone synthesized and stored in the anterior pituitary gland that stimulates milk) levels, it is often better to take blood before examination
- follicle-stimulating hormone (FSH) and luteinizing hormone (LH) estimation
- thyroid function tests, thyroid-stimulating hormone (TSH) and T4
- pelvic ultrasound examination to exclude polycystic ovaries and other abnormality. This may have to be transabdominal if vaginal examination is difficult.

An initial lead on the diagnosis may be given by raised FSH and LH levels (premature menopause), high prolactin levels (prolactinoma) or a raised LH:FSH ratio (polycystic ovaries). At this stage it is often preferable to refer the woman to an appropriate specialist. Women with polycystic ovaries are usually seen by a gynaecologist and those with other problems by an endocrinologist. Hirsuitism must be investigated as it is sometimes secondary to a virilizing tumour.

FSH, LH and serum oestradiol measured three times at three- to four-weekly intervals may be necessary to establish the diagnosis of early ovarian failure. Very high FSH, LH and low oestradial levels confirm a diagnosis of POF.

Chromosomal analysis is essential for all women under 30 years diagnosed with POF. A damaged or absent X chromosome occurs in Turner's syndrome and the presence of a Y chromosome is associated with a substantially increased risk of ovarian malignancy. Bilateral oophorectomy would be indicated if Y chromosomal material were found. This applies even to normal-looking women under 30 years. A geneticist would arrange this test (Davis 1996).

Tissue antibody screening can be arranged by a specialist department (gynaecology or endocrinology).

Physiological effects of amenorrhoea/ovarian failure may include loss of fertility, loss of bone density and increased risk of fractures, and increased risk of ischaemic heart disease (IHD). Reduced libido and possible vaginal dryness can affect sexual relationships. Psychological distress can result from premature menopause and its consequences or result from side effects of treatment or related conditions.

Aims of management

It is important to recognize the psychological impact of a diagnosis of premature menopause. Good doctor–patient communication, discussion and counselling are crucial at this stage. Once a diagnosis has been made, the following areas need to be considered:

- chromosome analysis
- hormone replacement therapy (HRT)
- type of HRT
    implant
    patches
    tablets
- management of interactions
    duration of treatment (long)
    monitoring
  ensuring continuation of therapy
- treatment of infertility in some women via ovum donation.

Bone mineral density estimation may be necessary in some cases. At the beginning of treatment, if postponement of HRT is being considered because of other medical problems or possible interactions, preliminary bone mineral density estimation will indicate if prophylactic treatment with biphosphonates should be prescribed.

Women with very early menopause may be too embarrassed to attend an HRT clinic and prefer to present to an ordinary surgery session where they can be referred to a dedicated clinic within the practice.

Communication breaking the news

For a young woman, the diagnosis of a premature menopause may feel catastrophic. The doctor needs to be sure of the diagnosis before communicating it and be aware of the sense of loss a woman feels when she knows that she can no longer bear children and that she is already postmenopausal and may perceive herself as 'old'. The images of youth and beauty which appear everywhere in the media encourage women to identify with them, so that to a certain extent the woman may feel she has lost her identity and cannot relate to her partner or friends as she did formerly. This loss of perceived status can also be damaging to a relationship, particularly if a couple were planning to start a family.

The doctor could approach the situation obliquely, as follows:

GP: Mary (first name), we have now got the results of the tests. Perhaps you know them already as you have been seeing the specialist (for women already referred to endocrinologist, etc.). The blood test shows that your ovaries have stopped working properly. This may be just a temporary problem. We're going to do another test in a few weeks and check how things are going.

Mary: Is this condition serious?

GP: This isn't a dangerous situation. You'll probably live to 82 and be perfectly well, but you would be advised to take hormone therapy. This puts back the oestrogen, the female hormone which your ovaries used to make.

Mary: Why do I need to take HRT? Doesn't it cause breast cancer?

GP: If you don't take it, the bones are likely to become fragile and you are more likely to have a fracture. Also, you are more at risk of heart disease. If you take HRT this keeps the bones strong and helps the heart.

Mary: What about breast cancer?

GP: About breast cancer – the increase in risk is very small. We all have a one in 12 risk of breast cancer and nobody can say whether you or I or anyone else will get it. HRT has a lot of advantages and in your case the advantages are likely to outweigh the risk. We're looking at quite a long period of HRT, at least until you're 50, but we'll monitor you very carefully and check you before you start treatment. There is a weekly clinic here, and the nurse and doctor will see you regularly to answer any questions.

Mary: Will I be able to start a family?

GP: At the moment your ovaries are not producing egg cells so you can't get pregnant. But we have a local clinic at...where they might be able to help you. There are a number of women in your situation, and the hospital has a system of giving you an egg donated by another woman which might be able to grow in your womb. This is done by in vitro fertilization.

The following list of questions appears in a booklet for women with premature menopause (*Health Alert* 1997):

* Is there a chance that my periods might start again?
* How long do I have to wait before knowing that they won't?
* What are the effects of an early menopause, both in the short and long term?
* What sort of treatment is available?
* Does it have any drawbacks?
* Are there any alternatives?
* What are my options if I want to have a child?
* Can you refer me to a specialist menopause clinic or an endocrinology clinic?
* How can I meet other women in my situation for support?

Psychological support

A dedicated clinic for menopausal women and HRT users may already be in place in the general practice and is the ideal solution for patients and practice teams (Coope & Roberts 1990; Roberts 1995). If the nurse and doctor can occupy parallel rooms, the workload is shared and many routine long-term HRT users may prefer to see the nurse, knowing that a doctor is available if necessary. Yearly monitoring can be incorporated into the repeat prescription computerized program as a request to see the doctor before the next prescription. A monitoring appointment need offer no more than a routine question: 'How are you?', and time allotted for discussion of length of treatment if requested, possible side effects, and weight or blood pressure measurement if due. The Ministry of Health circular (Department of Health 1998) recommends that routine breast examination does not form part of the monitoring, as a nurse can teach breast awareness at the initial screen.

The practice nurse is essential to the success of long-term HRT use, and prescription and training is now offered through the British Menopause Society (see Resources). Counselling about (IVF) in vitro fertilization and ovum donation is offered, if appropriate, through the relevant hospital department. Many practices now employ an attached clinical psychologist or counsellor (see Chapter 9 for discussion of egg donation).

Severe psychological stress may affect hypothalamic-pituitary-ovarian function adversely, although it does not cause POF. Sometimes women can be helped by individual counselling or sharing experiences within the context of a group (Harrison 1990) (see also Chapters 11 and 12).

Specific therapy for cause of amenorrhoea

Hypothyroidism (defined as a subnormal activity of the thyroid gland. In adult life it can cause mental and physical slowing, undue sensitivity to cold, slowing of the pulse, weight gain and coarsening of the skin (myxoedema)) is treated with thyroxine, and serial estimation of TSH, etc. may be needed to ensure that the dose is adequate. Interactions sometimes occur between HRT and thyroxine because oestrogen acts on the liver to increase thyroxine binding globulin (Ain et al. 1987).

Case study

> Margaret, aged 35, had a hysterectomy and both ovaries removed at 33 years for adhesions following endometriosis. She started HRT but felt ill, depressed and gained weight. Hypothyroidism was discovered a year later, but she still felt unwell on thyroxine treatment. She preferred to defer HRT until correct dose of thyroxine was reached and this was increased to 100 ug (micrograms) daily. We arranged repeat thyroid function tests and bone density estimation – if this was low, adequate prophylaxis of osteoporosis could be prescribed.

Hyperprolactinaemia

Bromocriptine and quinagolide are highly effective in the treatment of prolactinoma. However, there are side effects, which include nausea, vomiting and psychoses. Treatment needs to be given at night with food to reduce side effects, gradually increasing the dose. Serial prolactin levels are required to monitor the dose.

Polycystic ovary syndrome

Clomiphene is often given under gynaecological supervision to induce ovulation in women with polycystic ovary syndrome. It is an anti-oestrogen and may induce hot flushes.

Treatment of premature menopause

A wide choice of hormone treatments is available and decisions about HRT are best made jointly between the doctor and the woman. For women who decide to use HRT, it is essential to give enough oestrogen to prevent loss of bone density and control flushes and sweats. Women with a uterus may need added progestogen

10–12 days per 28 day cycle (Beresford et al. 1997). For most women, the minimum dose of HRT for prevention of osteoporosis is oral oestradiol 1–2 mg daily, conjugated equine oestrogen 0.625 mg daily or a 50 ug oestradiol patch. However, in young women a much higher dose is often necessary to control symptoms.

After a bilateral oopherectomy the gynaecologist may insert an implant of oestradiol β 50 mg and testosterone 50–100 mg. Testosterone can be highly effective in treating loss of libido which occurs after removal of ovarian androgens. One of the drawbacks of implants includes the impossibility of removal should side effects occur and the problem of tachyphylaxis. Symptoms may recur before the implant is due for renewal and an estimation of serum oestradiol shows that the level is still supra-physiological. This occurs because symptoms are manifested due to falling levels of circulating oestrogen, not the absolute level (Gangar et al. 1989).

It is often useful to have a gradual withdrawal from implants by the use of high-dose oestradiol patches. One of our patients needed two simultaneously applied 100 ug patches, supplemented with oestrogen gel. Vaginal oestrogen cream may also be necessary. The dose can be slowly reduced over the years. Transdermal oestrogen is chemically identical to oestradiol B used in implants and absorption is better than with the oral preparations. It is worth experimenting to find the right preparation for the individual.

Annual supervision at a dedicated clinic plus ad hoc consultations with the doctor or nurse can provide the necessary ongoing monitoring of treatment and changing of prescription if required. Side effects are common and include swelling of the breasts and tender nipples, weight gain in a few women and 'pre-menstrual' symptoms such as lethargy, headaches and depression during the progestogen phase of treatment. Libido may be reduced on oestrogen-only therapy and testosterone depot injections can be given for a few weeks to 'kick-start' sexual interest if needed. When these are established there may be no further need of testosterone medication.

Women with previous endometriosis may have this condition reactivated by HRT. They need specialist referral and prescription of continuous oestrogen and progesterone may be indicated to avoid triggering bleeding in the remaining endometriotic tissue.

Interaction between oestrogen and other medications can have serious consequences and may necessitate postponement or discontinuation of HRT. In such instances, alternative provisions need to be made to prevent osteoporosis, such as prescriptions of biphosphonates or calcium plus vitamin D3.

Women with a premature menopause who are also asthmatic, and dependent on corticosteroid medication, may find that control of asthma is lost. They need increased doses of cortiscosteroids to prevent severe breathlessness and wheezing (Lieberman et al. 1995). Oestrogen acts on the liver to increase production of sex hormone-binding globulin (Anderson 1974) and also thyroxine-binding and cortisol-binding globulins. If the binding globulin is increased, this diminishes the level of free-circulating cortisol and the woman should take larger doses of corticosteroids (Moore et al. 1978; Mashchak et al. 1982).

Case study

A woman of 43 had taken high doses of prednisolone from the age of 30. When she began HRT the asthma worsened and she was obliged to increase the dose of corticosteroids. Slight injuries to the legs resulted in tearing of the skin, with bleeding and the formation of ulcers. Eventually she ceased to take the oestrogen and the corticosteroids could be reduced to prednisolone 5 mg daily plus inhaled preparations. The ulcers healed and did not recur.

The side effects of high-dose corticosteroids include cataracts, delayed wound healing and diabetes. These may be sufficiently serious to justify withdrawal of HRT even in women with a premature menopause. In such cases, alternative measures should be taken to protect bone density (see Chapter 10). Serial measurements of bone density may be required.

Hypothyroidism

If a woman with a premature menopause also has myxoedema and is taking thyroxine, e.g. 100 ug daily, she may find that she feels ill after starting HRT. This is due to the increase in thyroxine-binding globulin (TBG), which binds thyroxine and decreases circulating free thyroxine. Urgent laboratory estimation of thyroid function is needed, with exploration of the clinical problem and current medication. It may be necessary to stop or postpone HRT until the situation is clarified. Local vaginal oestrogen creams or an oestrogen ring can be used as these do not affect liver function.

Bone density estimation

This is extremely useful in cases where a decision has to be made as to the desirability of using HRT. If bone mineral density is within the normal range for the woman's age, and she is a non-smoker, it is acceptable to postpone hormone treatment. If bone mineral density is reduced, other measures need to be taken to prevent osteoporosis. Bone density should be measured again at an appropriate interval to facilitate a decision on long-term treatment (WHO 1996).

The use of HRT and other treatments

Hormone therapy is the main medical treatment for women with a premature menopause. Contraindications include:

- breast cancer (previous or present)
- history of breast cancer before menopause in a sister or mother
- thromboembolism (defined as the condition in which a blood clot (thrombus), formed at one point in the circulation, becomes detached and lodges at another point), present active
- post-thromboembolism, especially if unprovoked. Refer to specialist laboratory to check if adverse clotting mechanisms are present
- some cases of endometriosis
- some cases of uterine/ovarian malignancy
- some cases of gall bladder disease/pancreatitis (Boston Collaborative Drug Surveillance Program 1974)
- severe liver or kidney disease. This limits metabolism and excretion of oestrogen.

Nearly all these are not absolute contraindications and the situation is usually resolved by referral and discussion with the appropriate specialist. Trials are now in progress to study the effects of HRT in breast cancer sufferers, particularly for the control of flushes secondary to tamoxifen (Powles et al. 1994; Marsden & Sacks 1997). So far the results are encouraging and survival has not been shortened in the group taking HRT compared with matched controls (Powles et al. 1993). The IBIS trial has been designed to measure the incidence of breast cancer in close relatives of women with breast cancer, with or without tamoxifen, in which some of the participants are taking tamoxifen (Denton 1995). To exclude the presence of breast cancer in women who are about to start hormone therapy, it may be necessary to examine the breasts. A recent circular from the Department of Health (1998) recommends that breasts should not be examined routinely but a nurse should teach breast awareness to women. Anxious women and those with symptoms should be offered examination. Mammography is not a 'must' for prescribing HRT, although in some countries it forms part of the initial assessment. Women with a lump are referred immediately for investigation. Ultrasound examination is often preferred to radiography in women under 40, because of increased vascularity of the breasts.

Present active thromboembolism may be made worse by oestrogen and some studies have demonstrated adverse coagulation changes on HRT (Coope et al. 1975; Poller et al. 1977). Four epidemiological studies have shown that venous thrombosis and pulmonary embolism are more common in women taking HRT than in non-users (Daly et al. 1996; Grodstein et al. 1996; Jick et al. 1996; Gutthan et al. 1997). The woman may be advised to postpone HRT until the situation is resolved by referral to an appropriate laboratory to check full blood count, fibrinogen protein C and S, prothrombin time and antithrombin III.

Recent myocardial infarction (which occurs when a segment of heart muscle ceases functioning after interruption of its blood supply) would be a contraindication because of the increased risk of pulmonary embolism. A recent trial of nearly 3000 women with coronary artery disease randomly allocated to HRT or placebo, showed that over four years, cardiovascular deaths were not reduced on active treatment, but thromboembolism and biliary disease increased (Hulley et al. 1998). Since the 1950s there has been published evidence that a premature menopause is associated with an increased risk of ischaemic heart disease (IHD) and atherosclerosis (a disease of the arteries that leads to restricted blood flow) (Witteman et al. 1989). Epidemiological studies show reduced risk of coronary heart disease in current users of HRT after the menopause (Stampfer et al. 1991). Whether women undergoing a major operation should stop HRT pre-operatively is a matter for consultation between the surgeon, anaesthetist and GP to advise the woman accordingly.

Endometriosis may flare up on HRT even if the ovaries and uterus have been removed. If this occurs, women may need referral to a gynaecologist. It is possible to give continuous progestogen and oestrogen (as in the combined oral contraceptive given continuously to young women) to women over 50 who still experience the long-term effects of a premature menopause. Kliofem, Elleste continuous or Premique may be prescribed.

Severe gall bladder disease may contraindicate HRT:

Case history

A woman of 40 developed severe osteoporosis, which was diagnosed on X-ray of the spine and which showed six compression fractures. She was treated with HRT and developed severe abdominal pain and vomiting. A computerized tomography (CT) scan showed multiple gallstones. Later she was admitted to hospital with acute pancreatitis. HRT was permanently contraindicated in this patient, who was prescribed alendronate and later vitamin D and calcium to preserve bone density.

A recent study of women under 60 years found that alendronate prevented bone loss to nearly the same extent as a combination of oestrogen and progestogen (Hosking et al. 1998). This may be a viable option for women with endometriosis and premature menopause.

Case history

Jane developed severe dysmenorrhoea in her teens and at first this was labelled by the doctors as 'all in the mind'. Eventually at the age of 25 she consulted a gynaecologist and endometriosis was diagnosed. She underwent an operation to remove fibroids. She was treated with danazol 100 mg three times a day, stopped treatment to try and conceive, and when this was unsuccessful, continued to take it for a total of 10 years. Periods became irregular with amenorrhoea of up to six months. At the age of 37, laparoscopy showed atrophic ovaries and extensive endometriotic scarring of the tubes. FSH and LH estimation showed postmenopausal levels. Her periods stopped altogether at age 40. She found it difficult to accept her infertility but coped well, developing interests such as charitable work and helping in the community. Premature menopause was diagnosed and she was treated with Prempak C, which caused severe cyclic pain and flaring up of endometriosis. Quantitative CT showed normal spinal bone mineral density. She stopped HRT and gave up smoking.

Jane's mother had developed breast cancer aged 46 and an aunt ovarian cancer, so Jane was referred to the local Family History Clinic, as she might have inherited the BRCAI gene. Mammography and intravaginal ultrasound were normal, but investigation of family history and CA 125 blood test showed that her risk of breast cancer is 40% and ovarian cancer 30%. Further quantitative CT of the spine showed reduction of bone density by a standard deviation of 1.4. HRT is contraindicated and she is being treated with Didronel PMO and Ovestin vaginal cream.

Continual supervision has been arranged with vaginal ultrasound and annual mammography. Prophylactic bilateral oophorectomy is being carried out in the near future and bilateral mastectomy is a possibility.

In all cases where premature menopause is complicated by the presence of other major disease or drug interaction which may contraindicate the use of HRT, alternative therapy should be offered, such as etidronate, alendronate, vitamin D + calcium and Livial, where these are not contraindicated by, for example, hypercalcaemia due to carcinomatous deposits, renal failure or severe oesophagitis. Livial (tibolone) 5 mg daily controls menopausal symptoms and probably does not affect recurrence of breast cancer. It preserves bone density and does not cause thrombophlebitis but there is no evidence that it is cardioprotective (Ginsburg & Prelevic 1995; Ginsburg et al 1995).

Many women with POF are at an age when their contemporaries are using oral contraceptives. It may be more acceptable to use continuous low-dose oral contraceptives than HRT. These can be effective in preserving bone mass (Barlow 1996).

Selective oestrogen modulators (SERMS) such as raloxifene have been shown to preserve bone density and do not stimulate the endometrium or breast in controlled trials (Delmas et al. 1997). Raloxifene is appropriate as a possible treatment for breast cancer patients with premature menopause. It has beneficial effects on blood lipids but does not control menopausal symptoms.

Timing of treatment

Although symptoms may be distressing there is no immediate urgency to treat until an informed decision has been made as to the best course of investigation and therapy. Significant loss of bone density does not occur overnight: it is important to disentangle the various strands of evidence in women with multiple diagnoses. If possible, the commencement of HRT should follow within a couple of weeks of diagnosis of premature menopause or oophorectomy. Women are usually encouraged to take it until the date at which a mid-life menopause would have occurred, i.e. age 50 (WHO 1996). It is helpful to provide women with written information about HRT and the reasons for taking it (prevention of fractures and heart disease, preservation of vaginal tissues, treatment of flushes and sweats, and secondary sleep disturbance). Duration of treatment needs to be discussed at the first prescription and thereafter, probably at yearly check-ups and again at age 50. The evidence that there is an increased risk of breast cancer over five years' use implies that duration of treatment may be questioned after five years (Beral 1997). The doctor and nurse need to be aware of unspoken anxieties, which may need to be aired, and time should be allocated for adequate counselling. However, doctors and nurses should also be aware of evidence that removal of the ovaries in young women reduces overall risk of breast cancer and that in those women with proven breast cancer, HRT has not been shown to shorten life (Bergkvist et al. 1989).

Continuation of treatment

The major problem with long-term HRT is non-compliance. The term 'compliance' is now regarded as unnecessarily authoritarian and perhaps paternalistic. 'Continuance' or 'adherence' have now been substituted, but the problem remains the same. Whichever term is used, the importance of continuing treatment cannot be overemphasized. HRT for over five years for prevention of osteoporotic fractures and current use to prevent cardiovascular disease are the essential points about treatment at any age (Stampfer et al. 1991). The danger is that women who agree to have long-term therapy may stop treatment without informing their doctor. An American study found that 30% of patients did not even cash the first prescription (Ravnikar 1987). A recent audit of prescriptions of HRT in the UK found that the highest rate of drop-out was in the first year of therapy. Reasons for stopping included weight gain and anxiety about cancer (Coope & Marsh 1992; Hope & Rees 1995).

Reasons for discontinuing HRT treatment

Anxiety about cancer, weight gain, bleeding problems, side effects and interactions of therapy are the main reasons for discontinuing therapy (Coope & Marsh 1992). Many of these difficulties can be surmounted by providing adequate initial diagnosis and assessment, an ongoing dedicated clinic for monitoring therapy, informing the other members of the practice team about vulnerable groups and availability of a specialized clinic for within-practice referrals.

Older women who experienced premature menopause are eligible for treatment at any age, and the PEPI (1996) study showed that

HRT use after the age of 55 years is effective in preserving bone density.

General practice is the only discipline equipped to identify the vulnerable groups and provide long-term monitoring and supervision of women with a premature menopause. Involvement and education of the whole primary care team is essential if women are to receive adequate treatment.

When to stop treatment

This is a difficult question and there are mixed views. Some suggest that for women with a premature menopause, treatment should be lifelong. However, many women would prefer to have repeated discussions on the basis of the most recent evidence of risks and benefits of HRT, especially with reference to their early loss of ovarian function and fear of cancer.

Individual risk/benefit assessment is necessary and this may be part of the initial screening and counselling. It may also follow the occurrence of a major illness or side effect, or be requested after a media scare about HRT.

Stopping oestrogen is always followed by flushes, even in those women who did not originally experience flushes before starting therapy. The occurrence of severe flushes may be a serious inconvenience to a woman who then feels she 'needs' treatment and in some cases she may fear that she is 'addicted' to HRT. Reduced doses of oestrogen may make withdrawal more gradual.

Rigorous assessment of risks and benefits should underlie the decision as to whether to continue with treatment. If the doctor feels it necessary to stop, as for instance in a case of pulmonary embolism, sympathetic counselling and support will usually suffice. It may be necessary to request specialist advice, as in this case, where anticoagulants plus HRT may be a possible course of action.

Case history

A woman taking long-term HRT attended the surgery with increasing breathlessness. Clinical examination was negative apart from mild hypertension. She was investigated with electrocardiogram (ECG), chest X-ray and detailed tests of pulmonary function. No cause was found until after several months a ventilation perfusion scan disclosed a large filling defect in the left lung field – a pulmonary embolism, which had been triggered by long-haul flights. She discontinued HRT.

Follow-up and monitoring

Many women are lost to follow-up and stop taking treatment unless arrangements are made to ensure continuity of positive supervision. Long-term therapy is particularly important for women with a premature menopause. Audit of HRT users in our practice found that it was possible to achieve nearly 90% adherence with therapy from one year to the next (Table 7.1), but even so this would imply that only 50% of these would be taking it after five years.

Table 7.1: Compliance

Year	Total number staying on HRT	Number users with uterus	Number hysterecto-mized users	Number stopping HRT in that year	Compliance = number staying on HRT expressed as % of number taking HRT at start of year
1986/87	88	29	59 (67%)	17	84%
1987/88	143	71	72 (50%)	18	89%
1988/89	246	125	121 (49%)	21	92%
1989/90	284	148	136 (48%)	45	86%
1990/91	260	130	130 (50%)	51	84%

From Coope & Marsh (1992). Reproduced with the permission of the author and publisher.

Provision of a dedicated nurse/doctor clinic is popular with patients (Roberts 1995) and we provide weekly parallel clinics with additional input in other surgery sessions. Referral from other doctors in the group practice ensures that complex cases and vulnerable patients are not missed and a high level of expertise can be maintained in a specialized area of knowledge.

Follow-up three months after the first prescription is essential so that the initial treatment can be altered and adjusted to suit the woman. It may be necessary to change the treatment several times until she reaches a satisfactory long-term regimen.

If bone density has been critical in the initial assessment before prescription, a bone scan will probably need to be repeated, perhaps in two to three years, to ensure that therapy is effective. Also, if circumstances change bone mineral density (BMD) measurement will help the decision on further treatment. Dual energy X-ray absorptiometry (DEXA) is preferable to quantitative CT because of the lower dose of radiation, convenience and rapidity of the test, and the large database, which ensures accuracy of comparison of results with women of similar age.

Community pharmacists could be involved routinely in the monitoring of HRT if there was better liaison with the primary healthcare team and mutually agreed protocols. Counselling rooms or space might need to be provided. A project is in progress in conjunction with the Northwick Park Hospital Menopause Unit to identify roles for the practice nurse and community pharmacist to aid GPs with organizing monitoring of women on HRT (Tanna & Pitkin 1997).

Women's needs alter with age. A young woman with premature menopause may have no problem with vaginal dryness at first, but gradually atrophic changes occur, which may necessitate local vaginal cream or an oestrogen-containing vaginal ring in addition to systemic therapy. Fertility is important to many young women and its loss may be experienced as catastrophic to a couple contemplating a family. Ovum donation is successful in 30% of referred cases. Shortage of eggs and lack of generosity in the expenses offered to donors under the law has resulted in long waits for treatment and 'private' referral may need to be considered. Contraception may appear inappropriate. However, in some rare cases, ovarian function may be resumed temporarily (Davis 1996). The use of barrier methods and specialist referral to a family planning clinic consultant may be helpful. The traditional advice is to wait two years before assuming infertility in a woman with amenorrhoea before age 50.

Case history

Frances, aged 30, found that her periods stopped for over 10 months and a pregnancy test was negative. She attended the surgery for diagnostic tests and assumed she was infertile. While awaiting the test results, she became pregnant. The couple were very dismayed at an unplanned pregnancy and requested a termination.

Health education

CHUSE to prevent osteoporosis

Calcium:	eat over 1 g daily
HRT:	discuss with doctor
Ultraviolet light:	over 15 minutes daily out doors
Smoking:	stop
Exercise:	weight-bearing good for bones, aerobic good for lungs and heart

The CHUSE aphorism has been used at our surgery as a poster in the waiting room and also at health education sessions. All these interventions have been shown by controlled trials and epidemiological studies to be effective in preventing osteoporosis and only one, HRT, involves financial expenditure – an import factor for budget-conscious women.

In general, smoking brings forward the timing of menopause (McKinlay et al. 1992b) and reduces levels of circulating oestrogen. It renders HRT less effective (Jensen et al. 1985; Krall & Dawson-Hughes 1991) and if symptoms persist in a woman who is taking a usually adequate dose of oestrogen, it is worth enquiring about her smoking habit. Cigarettes affect liver function and accelerate the metabolism/excretion of oestrogen. 'Old' skin is often apparent in the faces of heavy smokers. Persistent smokers who are apparently indifferent to its effect on the heart and lungs will often cut down or stop smoking if they learn about its reduction of circulating levels of oestrogen.

The health promotion approach for women can focus on the above as well as recommending strategies for healthy eating, increased physical activity and reducing smoking and blood pressure. Body mass index (BMI; weight in kilograms/height squared in metres) is relevant to bone density. Although some women are not eligible for HRT they should be informed that endogenous oestrogen is formed from adrenal hormones in their body fat, and this is a common source of oestrogen after the menopause. It is also a reason for not pursuing savage slimming diets.

There is strong evidence that a sedentary lifestyle increases the risk of coronary heart disease. Regular physical activity reduces low-density lipoprotein (LDL) levels, overweight and reduces blood pressure. Maintenance of regular physical activity is important for cardiovascular health and is protective against strenuous exercise acting as a trigger for a cardiovascular incident. Raised blood pressure has been shown to increase coronary heart disease, cardiac failure and stroke. Lifestyle changes that reduce blood pressure include reducing dietary salt intake, reduction in weight and alcohol use, and increased physical activity.

Organization of the practice to provide a service to women with premature menopause

To serve the needs of women with premature menopause, the practice should aim to identify three main vulnerable groups:

* bilateral oopherectomy before 50 years
* hysterectomy before 50 years with ovaries conserved
* early natural menopause.

Women who have both ovaries removed or irradiated before 50 years should have this entered on the practice computer. It should be possible to alert the partners to the possibility of hormone replacement therapy and check the patient's medication when she attends the surgery. Referral to the practice HRT clinic is arranged for those not taking HRT, when discussion, counselling and alternative medication can be offered to those unable or unwilling to take oestrogen. HRT remains the most effective and cheapest treatment (Francis et al. 1995).

Hysterectomy with the preservation of ovaries should be entered on the computer because of the awareness that premature ovarian failure sometimes follows (Watson & Studd 1993). This is not always the case, and a Danish study demonstrated normal bone density in such women compared with community controls (Ravn et al. 1995).

FSH estimation is essential to identify those who need early hormone replacement therapy (Seeley 1992). This is a cheap, non-invasive test that can be repeated every two or three years to ascertain the timing of menopause. The reason for postponing HRT until the FSH rises significantly is the increase in breast cancer incidence in long-term users. Most women would prefer to defer oestrogen therapy as long as possible until ovarian failure, when loss of bone density is most rapid.

Early natural menopause is identified when taking the history of the last menstrual period in women attending for cervical smear screening. The diagnosis can be put on computer and women can then be offered referral to the practice HRT clinic.

Vulnerable groups, such as long-term, high-dose thyroxine and corticosteroid users, women with personal or family history of early myocardial infarction, diabetic patients and those with hyperlipidaemia (the presence in the blood of an abnormally high concentration of fats) need to be targeted by the practice. If vulnerability is combined with a premature menopause, there is a strong case for treatment with HRT or alternative therapy (Coope & Coope 1996).

Vulnerable groups include:

- women with early (premenopausal) oophorectomy or ovarian irradiations
- women with hysterectomy before menopause
- long-term corticosteroid users
- long-term thyroxine users
- women with a family history of osteoporosis
- women with a body mass index <20 – found at women's health clinic
- women with a family history of early cardiac death
- women who already have:
     ischaemic heart disease (IHD)
     coronary artery bypass graft (CABG)
     positive coronary angiogram
     angina
- women with two or more raised risk factors for IHD:
     cholesterol > 7.0 mmol/l
     smoking > 15 cigarettes daily
     BP >160/90 mm Hg
- women with early fragility fracture, e.g. Colles fracture (a fracture of the lower end of the forearm just above the wrist, usually caused by a fall on the outstretched hand, named after Irish surgeon A Colles [1773–1843]) before 60 years).
- women with late fragility fracture, e.g. low trauma fracture need bone density measurement. If significantly reduced, consider HRT or biphosphonates.

Menopausal women with a history of early amenorrhoea are at high risk of osteoporosis (Davies et al. 1990), and this continues throughout their lives.

Guidelines for good practice

There is no published experimental evidence as to the best way of managing the menopause in general practice, apart from Roberts (1995) finding that women prefer a dedicated clinic. A consensus meeting of GPs at the annual British Menopause Society meeting in

Birmingham,1997 concluded that:

Supervision shared between doctor and nurse is preferable. This can be worked out in each practice but the negative attitude of The Royal College of Nursing towards breast examination by nurses implies that doctors examine breasts and nurses can teach breast awareness.

Definite contraindications to HRT are carcinoma of breast or endometrium. Possible contraindications include previous spontaneous thromboembolism. These patients should have clotting profile checked (antithrombin III, protein C and S) and be referred to a specialist clinic. Recent advice from the Medicines Control Agency suggests that HRT should stop pre-operatively but there is no general agreement and GPs should check with the individual surgeon and anaesthetist concerned. Endometriosis may be reactivated by HRT and may need to be discussed with the gynaecologist. Continuous combined therapy should be appropriate. Gall bladder disease may be worsened.

In the past other conditions have been wrongly considered as contraindications. None of the following contraindicates HRT: ischaemic heart disease, cardiac valve disease, long-term anticoagulation, hypertension, varicose veins, hyperc-holesterolaemia, hypertrigleyccridaemia, a family history of pre-menopausal breast cancer, benign breast disease, uterine fibroids, abnormal smears, malig-nant diseases that are not hormonally sensitive, diabetes mellitus, epilepsy, migraine, otosclerosis, osteoporosis, smokers and women over 60 years of age.

Figure 7.1 outlines the protocol for individual practices.

1 Contraindications to HRT should be excluded.
2 Counselling is needed for each woman on risks and benefits of HRT, length of use and pros and cons of breast cancer risk versus prevention of cardiovascular disease and osteoporosis.
3 History should be taken to ensure that the woman is menopausal. In case of doubt before 45 years two separate FSH blood tests six weeks apart: if either is over 30 u/l, the diagnosis is premature menopause. If in doubt, refer to a specialist.
4 Contraception should be discussed. For sexually active women who have not been sterilized, it is needed in the perimenopause, and also one year post-menopause if over 50 years, two years postmenopause if less than 50 years old. It should be claimed for on GMS4. Exclude pregnancy as a cause of amenorrhoea.
5 Check breasts and teach breast awareness. Remind of importance of accepting three-yearly mammography screen.
6 Record blood pressure.
7 Vaginal examination within the year of commencing HRT. Abnormal bleed-ing or findings on examination need referral.
8 Discuss choice of preparation.
9 Short-term side effects are explained.

Figure 7.1: Individual practice protocols. Reproduced with permission of *Journal of British Menopause Society* (1997).

Advantages of a dedicated HRT/menopause/health promotion clinic include:

* scarce resources targeted on need
* nurse works to full potential and has medical back-up
* screening for cervical cancer
* nurse teaches breast self-examination
* family planning
* dietary advice
* variety of treatments offered to women
* continuous care and emotional support.

Conclusion

Women who have a premature menopause need to be especially aware of potential long-term health risks and what they can do to help themselves. Although there is concern for immediate relief from menopausal symptoms, and much can be done using lifestyle changes, every effort needs to be made to ensure good long-term health with the use of both conventional medicine and non-medical approaches. With personal involvement and long-term commitment, many women find it helpful to control aspects of their health and wellbeing using lifestyle changes. Above all, the focus of assessment and treatment should be patient-centred, that is, tailored to each individual woman's needs.

Chapter 8
Medical approaches to premature menopause in a gynaecological clinic

JOAN PITKIN AND CAROLYN ALLAN

Introduction

Menopause at a young age can be associated with significant short-term morbidity with regard to a woman's physical, psychological and sexual health. As women in this situation may spend up to 50% of their lives in a postmenopausal state, the increased long-term risks of cardiovascular disease and osteoporotic fractures resulting from hypo-oestrogenism (lowered oestrogen levels) are particularly significant.

Premature ovarian failure (POF) represents one of the most demanding aspects of menopausal care for the clinician (Abernethy 1997a). Often women with premature menopause find it difficult to fully accept the situation. They may have been career-oriented and delayed having a family, never dreaming that their fertility may be lost prematurely and permanently. For others, premature menopause may follow a variety of clinical scenarios. These include prolonged pelvic pain, which is itself secondary to pelvic inflammatory disease; or endometriosis, possibly leading to bilateral oophorectomy; or it may result from chemo- or radiotherapy for a number of both malignant and non-malignant indications. Women who have undergone a surgical menopause experience a rapid and dramatic fall in their endogenous oestrogen levels. This can result in extremely uncomfortable vasomotor symptoms, which can cause greater anxiety and distress than that experienced by women for whom the onset of menopause was a more gradual physiological process.

Although hypogonadotrophic hypogonadism (cessation of gonadal function as a result of low luteinizing hormone [LH] and follicle-stimulating hormone [FSH] levels does not in itself represent primary failure of ovarian function, women with amenorrhoea due to pituitary or hypothalamic dysfunction, including weight-related amenorrhoea, will also be represented in the group of early onset oligo- (infrequent periods) or amenorrhoeic (no periods) women who are referred to a gynaecological clinic for management of their hypo-oestrogenism.

Initial assessment and screening

A full history is taken and a thorough physical examination, including pelvic examination, with cervical smear if indicated, is performed at the first visit. Climacteric symptoms will be documented with the aid of a formal symptom score chart or visual analogue scale. Women with idiopathic (unexplained) premature menopause may have a positive family history of early ovarian failure, with an odds ratios of as high as 6:1 reported, although recall bias may partly explain this (Torgerson et al. 1997). Smoking has also – controversially – been associated with premature menopause, although when seeing women in the menopause clinic the relevance of a history of cigarette smoking is used primarily to assess cardiovascular risk. A detailed review of the other recognized cardiovascular risk factors is carried out and a baseline lipid profile, including low and high density cholesterol and triglyceride measurements, is obtained. At present screening for the atherosclerosis (a condition in which fatty plaques develop on the inner walls of the artery, which eventually can restrict blood flow) predisposition gene is only available in a research setting.

Alternative causes of amenorrhoea, such as thyrotoxicosis (a condition due to excessive amounts of thyroid hormones in the bloodstream, which can cause a rapid heartbeat, sweating, tremor and anxiety, among other symptoms) and hyperprolactinaemia (the overproduction of the hormone prolactin, levels of which control lactation), need to be excluded with thyroid function tests and serum prolactin levels respectively (see also Chapter 7). Serial FSH levels may be required to document sustained hypergonadotrophic hypogonadism.

The role of ovarian biopsy and ultrasound for follicle detection, and the place of detailed immunological and endocrinological investigations to delineate cases of autoimmunity and ovarian resistance have been discussed in Chapter 2.

Documentation of a full past medical and surgical history is important as it will influence what, if any, hormonal therapy is to be offered. It is important to use this initial consultation to build up a complete picture of the individual woman's risk-benefit profile for hormone replacement therapy (HRT) in order to assess how best to serve her interests and to accurately advise as to how long she might need to continue with the treatment.

A woman may be at particular risk of osteoporosis because of previous or current corticosteroid therapy which she has received or is receiving as part of the treatment for the condition underlying the onset of POF. Other risk factors, such as smoking, caffeine intake and poor exercise levels, are softer indicators of decreased bone density. All women with premature menopause should be offered formal bone densitometry studies to estimate current risk and to establish a baseline for treatment. Calcanial ultrasonography is currently being evaluated as an alternative technique, at least for initial screening. Uncertainty still surrounds the use of bone markers and at present their use is limited; they are most helpful in following response to treatment.

Breast screening is one of the most controversial areas of management of women receiving HRT. It is increasingly accepted that mammography is useful for screening in the over-40 age group whereas in the past it was reserved for women 50 years and over. Nevertheless, breast tissue is really too dense for accurate mammographic assessment below the age of 40 and in this group breast ultrasonography is more beneficial. There has been much controversy about the increased density of breast tissue subsequent to the ingestion of HRT (Stomper et al. 1990). Laya and colleagues (1996) reported that there is an increased incidence of interval breast malignancies in HRT users compared with non-users, presumably indicating that small early breast tumours had been missed on mammographic assessment in the hormone-treated group due to oestrogen-induced increased breast density. However, this was a small group of women, and in America annual screening is common. Other studies have noted that age is an important determinant of the risk of a diagnosis of an interval cancer. In England and Holland the incidence is highest in the age group below 60 years, which is where the uptake of HRT is highest and this is where the American observations may link in. In the future, women may be advised to discontinue HRT for a short period of time before mammography to allow more accurate screening. At present, however, there is insufficient information to be able to advise women as to how long they would need to discontinue treatment prior to their breast screening or how long it takes for the breast tissue to return to 'normal' pre-treatment levels. Other screening modalities, e.g. magnetic resonance imaging (MRI) breast screening, are still under investigation.

The clinician needs to approach this scenario with immense sensitivity and understanding. These women will often need several visits to come to terms with the issues involved. It is important to bear in mind that no harm will come to them immediately, although the vasomotor symptoms, if present, may cause considerable reduction in quality of life. Long-term outcomes are potentially associated with a reduction in the quality of life and can be life threatening and discussions about therapy should clearly outline this.

Treatment options

When evaluating a young woman who has experienced a premature menopause, there are a number of points to be considered with regard to treatment. If there is any doubt about the diagnosis or if the patient is oligomenorrhoeic (has infrequent periods) rather than amenorrhoeic (no periods), i.e. she is perimenopausal, then fertility cannot be assumed to be irreversibly lost. Any treatment strategy must include contraceptive cover if the woman does not desire pregnancy. Then there are the wishes of the woman herself. Given that the basic obligation of therapy is reoestrogenization to protect against the short- and long-term effects of premature menopause on her health, the woman may prefer to opt for the contraceptive pill simply because it appears more 'natural' for a woman of her age to carry the pill rather than a HRT packet in her handbag. This may assist in preventing her feeling isolated from other women in her peer group. On this regimen she will menstruate regularly and, in the circumstances described above, will have the necessary contraceptive cover.

The oestrogenic component of HRT may be administered in a number of different formulations (see Tables 8.1 and 8.2). Of these, oral is the most widely prescribed. Women, particularly those who may already be taking oral medication, are often quite content to take an oral hormone preparation because of the convenience, and as they have already established a daily routine, adherence should not be an issue. Those women who have become menopausal as a result of medical or surgical interventions will probably have already taken, or still be taking, oral treatment for other health problems.

Table 8.1: Components of hormone replacement therapy and related preparations

Oestrogens
- conjugated equine oestrogens (CEE)
- 17 β oestradiol
- oestradiol valerate
- oestrone

Progestogens
- progesterone
- progesterone analogues (C-21 derivatives)
    dydrogesterone
    medroxyprogesterone acetate

Testosterone analogues (19 nor-testosterone derivatives)
- norethisterone/norethisterone acetate
- levonorgestrel

Gonadomimetics
- tibolone

Selective oestrogen receptor modulators (SERMs)
- raloxifene

Table 8.2: Routes of administration

Oestrogen
- oral
- transdermal
    patch
    gel
- implant
- vaginal preparations
    cream
    pessary
    ring

Progestogens
Progesterone
- oral
- vaginal
    gel
    pessary
Progesterone analogues (C-21 derivatives)
- oral

Testosterone analogues (19 nor-testosterone derivatives)
- oral
- transdermal (as combined therapy)

Gonadomimetics
- oral

SERMs
- oral

An important consideration when choosing the most appropriate form of oestrogen is the possibility of oestrogen sensitivity, which is suggested by a history of severe gestation-related nausea, i.e. hyperemesis (abnormally severe vomiting in pregnancy), cyclical breast pain or fluid retention either during pregnancy or when on the contraceptive pill. Some women will find that one natural oestrogen is better tolerated than another and a process of trial and error may identify a suitable alternative. For others a non-oral oestrogen may be better tolerated, such as transdermal patches, gel or implants. Symptoms referable to urogenital atrophy, such as painful intercourse, dysuria (painful or difficult urination) and urgency, will usually respond to locally administered, non-systemically absorbed preparations. Such vaginal preparations are usually only prescribed in circumstances where systemic oestrogens are best avoided (see below).

Personal inclinations also need to be taken into account. Gels may be seen to 'normalize' the situation as the woman may view this as akin to using body lotion, being more 'cosmetic' than therapeutic. The oestrogen gel is applied daily but must be used in combination with progestogen, delivered as a tablet in the non-hysterectorized woman. The issue here is that some women may forget or deliberately not take the progestogen tablets and it is therefore wise to carefully monitor who is most likely to adhere to treatment, otherwise the clinician is inadvertently prescribing unopposed oestrogen. Transdermal patches are equally as efficacious as oral compounds in alleviating the short-term effects of hypo-oestrogenism and offer comparable bone protection. They have a theoretical advantage over oral preparations in terms of their effect on triglyceride levels, insulin sensitivity and lack of predisposition to gallstone formation (Chetkowski et al. 1986; Cheang et al. 1994). Some women, however, reject the concept of a transdermal patch because they are resistant to the idea of being 'labelled'. The comment is frequently made that they do not wish their partner to see the patch and several admit to removing the patch before making love and reapplying it afterwards.

Finally, oestrogen may be taken in the form of an implant. This is a very successful and practical way of administering long-term oestrogen if adequately monitored. It also has the advantage of allowing administration of concomitant testosterone replacement (see below). There is one disadvantage with the oestrogen implant. Although it is ideal for hysterectomized women, for women who still require endometrial protection there is again a need to take 12 to 14 days of progestogen tablets per month, and this treatment may need to be continued for some time after the oestrogen implants have been withdrawn, as circulating levels can remain high for a significant period of time. The delivery of oestrogen as an implant has several advantages. It allows a slightly higher level of serum oestradiol to be achieved, which is often necessary in the younger woman for symptom control. Once stabilized, it is usually unnecessary to repeat implants more than six-monthly and often women do not need implants for nine months, which makes it both convenient and trouble-free. However, there are problems with this delivery system, namely: the accumulation of multiple small scars, the need to attend a surgery or clinic on a regular basis, and the issue of continuing ingestion of progestogen. The most widespread concern, however, is that of tachyphylaxis (the development of the need for supraphysiological levels of oestrogen such that increasing doses are required to maintain the desired effect). In this scenario, a woman adjusts to supraphysiological levels of oestrogen, making her particularly sensitive to the fall in oestrogen level rather than the absolute values. The result is that she is often drenched in sweats and flushes while having serum oestradiol levels of over 2000 pmol/l. Such a situation can be avoided if regular oestradiol levels are taken prior to implant insertion. Levels are best maintained within the range of 800 to 1200 pmol/l.

Use of testosterone as part of a postmenopausal hormone replacement regimen remains controversial. It is particularly worth considering in women who have undergone bilateral oophorectomy because of the associated 50% fall in their circulating androgens. Women, particularly those who experience early loss of ovarian function, may continue to suffer from reduced sexual desire or libido despite adequate oestrogenization. At a dose of 50 mg subcutaneously every six months, testosterone does not appear to adversely effect lipid profiles and does not lead to virilization (Burger & Davis 1998). Reoestrogenization itself will relieve poor libido occurring as a secondary phenomenon, relating to vaginal dryness and compounded by sweats and flushes, the so-called domino effect (Campbell & Whitehead 1977), and this should be addressed before testosterone replacement is considered.

A further oral alternative for women in whom libido is of particular concern is tibolone, a gonadomimetic with oestrogenic, progestogenic and androgenic characteristics. It has tissue-specific metabolism with a progestogenic effect on the endometrium and very little breast activity (Kloosterboer & Deckers 1997). It is effective in treating urogenital symptomatology. Because of its lack of endometrial stimulation it does not result in a withdrawal bleed. Some women do not respond as well in terms of their vasomotor symptoms, although in clinical trials it has been shown it to be as efficacious as sequential combined therapy (Hammar et al. 1998).

When choosing a suitable hormone replacement regimen for a woman, regardless of age, it is also important to elicit any tendency to progestogen sensitivity. Women with a history of severe premenstrual tension or side effects during the progestogenic phase of the combined oral contraceptive pill are likely to have a progestogen sensitivity. In these situations, it is important to choose a regimen with a mild progestogen rather then one of the more androgenic 19 nor-testosterone derivatives. Some women will find that even the C-21 derivatives, e.g. dydrogesterone and medroxyprogesterone acetate, cause side effects. Dydrogesterone, for example, can induce headaches. These women may be best incorporating a natural progesterone into their hormone replacement regimen. Natural progesterones are currently available as micronized progesterone suppositories and intravaginal gel. Unfortunately these modes of delivery are not universally popular. Oral micronized progesterone can only be obtained in the UK on a named patient basis, although it is readily available in other European countries and in the USA. As yet, there is no patch available that contains the milder C-21 derivative progestogens.

Selective (o)estrogen receptor modulators (SERMs) are a rapidly expanding class of drugs which, as their name suggests, interact with the oestrogen receptor, but with differing affinity and specificity to the various oestrogen responsive tissues (Delmas et al. 1997). This family of drugs developed from the observation that tamoxifen had oestrogenic effects on endometrium and bone and anti-oestrogenic effects on breast. Work is continuing to develop highly specific compounds and this is likely to significantly improve our ability to tailor therapy to the individual woman's needs, particularly with respect to the breast cancer issue, as there is some evidence to suggest that raloxifene will not increase the risk and may in addition have a protective effect (Cummings et al. 1999). However, long-term data are still needed. We have highlighted the current and potential future roles of SERMs with regard to bone and cardiovascular protection (lipid-lowering effect) in the following section reviewing complex clinical cases. Of note, however, is the fact that they do not relieve vasomotor symptoms.

Finally, the so-called natural or alternative remedies, including phytoestrogens and wild yam, are still being evaluated in clinical trials. While the data on the progestogenic effect of the wild yam are not particularly promising, the increasing volume of literature pertaining to the oestrogenic effects of phytoestrogens suggests that they may well have a legitimate role in the management of the menopause (Tham et al. 1998). Phytoestrogens are plant-derived compounds that activate the oestrogen receptor. In cultures with a high phytoestrogen intake (e.g. Japan) the incidence of cardiovascular disease is lower in comparison with those societies where these foods are not as extensively consumed. Initial work also suggests a favourable effect of the isoflavanes, one of the two major classes of phytoestrogens in our diet, on bone. This work is still in its infancy and as such we cannot make recommendations about their role in managing the menopause, particularly premature menopause where ingestion would be long term. (For further discussion of phytoestrogens and non-medical approaches see Chapter 10.)

With the number of therapeutic options available, it behoves the clinician to spend some time outlining the alternatives to the woman concerned and involving her in the decision-making process. Indeed, if she does not play an active part at this time, there is a very real risk of adversely affecting her adherence to the therapy, and clearly the success of any treatment strategy is based on its long-term uptake. Commitment is of the utmost importance and this will only be obtained if the woman feels that she has been listened to, that she has been involved in planning and choosing the management strategy, and that she feels that the clinician has an understanding and an empathy for her situation.

If a woman opts for the contraceptive pill then it is reasonable to prescribe a third-generation progestogen pill. There was much controversy about these pills in 1995, with epidemiological evidence suggesting that they predisposed to venous thromboembolism to a greater degree than their second-generation progestogen counterparts. It was largely agreed, however, that they have a more favourable lipid profile. Latterly more evidence from the European collaboration study has suggested that there is no increased risk for venous thromboembolism (Spitzer 1997; Suissa et al. 1997). The third-generation combined oral contraceptive pills are the combined oral contraceptive of choice, as they tend not to be associated with mood swings and premenstrual tension, and are less likely to cause greasy skin, acneform rashes and fluid retention than the earlier generation contraceptive pills, predominantly because they are progestogen receptor-specific and have little interaction with androgen receptors.

If the woman prefers a non-synthetic oestrogen, but there remains concern about fertility, two options are available to her. A HRT regimen incorporating a daily progestogen-only pill with added progestogen for 14 days a month to protect the endometrium can be constructed or, alternatively, with the introduction of the Mirena progestogen-secreting coil, the endometrial protection can be ingested at source with the oestrogen taken in any form that the woman chooses: tablet, patch, gel or implant (Raudaskoski et al. 1995). As with any progestogen-based contraception there is at least a 30% chance of irregular bleeding for the first few cycles after the Mirena coil has been inserted, and eventually almost 30% of women are rendered amenorrhoeic. With prior counselling this does not appear to be a significant disincentive.

One of the key issues that must be discussed with the woman is whether or not she wishes to have a monthly bleed. Older post-menopausal women often elect to have a 'period-free' preparation, particularly if they have been amenorrhoeic for 12 months prior to commencing treatment. The younger woman, however, may elect to have a monthly bleed as she feels more akin to her peers. It is also possible to experience a withdrawal bleed on a three-monthly basis. Most importantly, assumptions should not be made as each woman will have her own reasons for choosing a particular regimen.

Complicated clinical scenarios

Systemic lupus erythematosus (SLE)

Women with systemic lupus erythematosus (SLE, often abbreviated to lupus erythematosus (LE), is a chronic inflammatory disease of connective tissue affecting the skin and various internal organs), who undergo treatment with pulse cyclophosphamide, face an increased risk of POF, with reported incidences of between 40% and 45% (McDermott & Powell 1996). Two-thirds of women who develop ovarian failure, determined by cessation of menstruation and confirmed by oestradiol and gonadotrophin levels, do so within two years of starting treatment. Factors that increase the risk of ovarian failure are age, duration and cumulative dose of treatment. The degree of bone marrow suppression achieved also appears to relate to the risk. In addition, women with lupus are quite likely to have received corticosteroid therapy at some time during the course of their illness. Prednisolone (or an equivalent corticosteroid) administered in doses greater than physiological replacement, 7.5 mg daily (or the dose equivalent), for extended periods is well-recognized as causing bone loss. This combination of chemotherapeutic insults therefore leads not only to early loss of ovarian function, with its adverse metabolic sequelae, but results in this group of women having two significant risk factors for the development of osteopaenia (early bone loss) and subsequently osteoporosis. Case reports linking POF directly to the underlying disease process itself have also been published (Case records of the Massachusetts General Hospital 1986).

The incidence of premature cardiovascular disease is increased in women with lupus. It is reported that the risk of myocardial infarction in patients in the 35–44 year age group is 50 times greater than that reported in women of a similar age in the Framingham Offspring Study (Manzi et al. 1997). An important factor in this increased risk is the presence of early ovarian failure. Prolonged corticosteroid usage is another contributory factor.

There are concerns about the use of HRT in this group of women because of the strong evidence linking sex steroids to the pathophysiologic process that leads to the development of SLE. This has been demonstrated in murine animal models (mice), in in vitro work and also in observational human studies showing both temporal relationships between exposure to oestrogen and development of lupus (Sanchez-Guerrero et al. 1995), and the significantly increased risk associated with the female gender: 6–8:1. However, small prospective and retrospective studies have not shown any increase in the rate or severity of disease flares in women taking oestrogen replacement therapy. A larger study addressing the safety of oestrogens in SLE (Safety of Estrogens in Lupus Erythematosus – National Assessment Trial) is currently underway in the UK.

Management of women in these situations is always complex and is best provided by the joint care of the rheumatology and menopause clinics. Women who have evidence of a phospholipid syndrome with the associated increased risk of thrombosis, will also need input from a specialist haematologist. In some cases, women will already be receiving anticoagulation therapy, and depending on the efficacy of the regimen used, this may need to be modified if oestrogen replacement is to be introduced. Other women may need to be anticoagulated in order to safely commence oestrogen therapy.

The choice of therapy for women with lupus and POF is dictated by how their illness manifests itself, by their short-term oestrogen deficiency symptoms and by their long-term osteoporosis and cardiovascular risk profiles. Baseline assessment should include, in addition to the routine screening described previously, formal bone densitometry and a full thrombophilia profile (if not already documented).

Women who present predominantly with the acute effects of oestrogen withdrawal are most likely to benefit from traditional oestrogen and progestogen replacement (if endometrial protection is required). There are theoretical benefits with the use of transdermal oestrogens because of their lack of effect on clotting parameters in comparison to oral preparations, although this has not been shown to affect the risk of venous thromboembolism, either in the general population or in women with a documented phospholipid syndrome. When considering which progestogen to use, the androgenic progestogens have a documented effect on improving bone density in their own right (Abdalla et al. 1985), although the non-androgenic progestogens have a more favourable lipid profile. The clinical scenario may well dictate which progestogen is most appropriate. There is certainly a potential role for the use of concomitant biphosphonate therapy with a lipid-friendly progestogen. If the woman does not suffer from the effects of acute oestrogen withdrawal then there may be a place for a SERM to preserve bone, although in a group of this age range the rate of subsequent vasomotor side effects may be unacceptable. Nevertheless, they may be a viable alternative especially if the lack of effect on an increase in the risk of breast cancer is shown to be true in long-term follow up studies. They do, however, carry the same increased venous thromboembolism risk as traditional HRT. If bone protection is the only significant indication for treatment then biphosphonates should be strongly considered, particularly if corticosteroid use is to be or has been prolonged.

Other non-hormonal alternatives for specific short- and long-term hypo-oestrogenic sequelae, as outlined in the section below, addressing breast cancer may be relevant, particularly if the woman has a prothrombotic tendency but has not had a complication of this and would not otherwise be anticoagulated.

It is important to remember in following these women over time that neither the manifestations of their lupus nor of their oestrogen deficiency are static, and that their evolution and continued codependence may alter both the indication for treatment and the framework within which hormone therapy is to be prescribed.

The fertility, emotional and psychological issues that accompany the premature loss of ovarian function have been dealt with elsewhere, and in this particular group of women, the compounding effect of these on the already distressing consequences of chronic illness must be seriously considered.

Breast cancer

As the number of women being diagnosed with breast cancer before their menopause increases, and the use of adjuvant chemotherapy (such as cyclophosphamide, methotrexate and flourouracil [CMF]) becomes more widespread, more women with malignant breast disease are experiencing a premature loss of ovarian function. Currently, 50% of women at presentation have curable disease, with approximately 25% expected to experience a recurrence. Forty to fifty per cent of women aged under 40 who receive adjuvant chemotherapy in the form of CMF will experience ovarian failure (Bines et al. 1996). Greater probability of long-term survival means that not only do these women have to contend with the short-term effects of oestrogen deprivation but that the cardiovascular and bone effects must also be taken into consideration.

The use of oestrogen replacement therapy in women surviving breast cancer was the subject of a recent consensus conference (Santen et al. 1998). Although there is a small amount of data from observational studies of oestrogen replacement therapy in breast cancer patients, at present there are no data from larger clinical trials. Until such information is available, oestrogen should only be considered when all other treatment options have been exhausted and, if used at all, it should be taken in the smallest dose possible for the shortest duration possible. After a full and frank discussion about the risk-benefit ratio, the final decision should be made by the woman herself, with the support of the supervising clinician. The role of combination tamoxifen and HRT treatment was also considered at this conference. While there are preliminary biochemical data to suggest a possible role for the administration of concomitant tamoxifen and low-dose oestrogen, there is no trial information about either the efficacy or the safety of this regimen.

Non-hormonal alternatives are dependent on the indication for treatment. Amelioration of vasomotor symptoms by approximately 25% is seen with placebo therapies. Clonidine and, less effectively, vitamin E, have a statistically greater effect than placebo but are less potent than oestrogen. Some antidepressants may also have a role to play in alleviating sweats and flushes. Megestrol acetate has also been shown to be effective but there remains concern about the effects of progestogens on the breast tissue. Urogenital atrophy will respond to the local application of non-absorbable oestrogens and there does not appear to be any appreciable rise in systemic oestrogen levels, although at commencement of treatment there may be absorption if the vaginal mucosa is particularly atrophic. More work is required to confirm this. Lubricants are less helpful. Some woman perceive this form of application of therapy to be less than ideal but with demonstration and encouragement many will be successful in its usage.

Biphosphonates are the treatment of choice for bone preservation in this group of women with both breast cancer and POF. It has been shown that such women are at increased risk of accelerated bone loss in comparison with their peers who maintain regular menstruation following chemotherapy (Headley et al. 1998). Several small studies have also shown a favourable effect on bone metastases and their complications with some of the bisphosphonates (Kanis et al. 1996). Tamoxifen itself acts as an oestrogen on bone, reversing the loss that is seen with placebo but there are no data about possible reduction of fracture risk. The results of trials currently underway involving raloxifene are of great importance to these women, who require cardiovascular and bone protection without putting them at increased risk of relapse or recurrence of their breast disease. Importantly, SERMs such as raloxifene do not have the stimulatory effect on the endometrium seen with tamoxifen (Delmas et al. 1997).

As these women continue to have an improved life expectancy, their cardiovascular profile assumes increasing importance. At present, it is recommended that therapeutic strategies focus on non-hormonal alternatives, in particular the class of drugs known as statins, 3-hydroxy-3-methylglutaryl coenzyme A reductase inhibitors. These have been shown to reduce low-density and total cholesterol levels and to reduce cardiovascular morbidity and mortality in both primary and secondary prevention trials. Again

SERMs may have a role in the future as they too appear to favourably modulate lipid profiles, but more data are required. However neither SERMs nor statins demonstrate the direct effect on vasculature that oestrogen does (Collins 1996). Advising women about the risks of cardiovascular disease versus breast cancer relapse or recurrence is an emotive issue and results from prospective randomized clinical trials are badly needed, for example, the Women's Health Initiative (Mathews et al. 1997).

CASE ILLUSTRATION

A subgroup of women may have genuine concerns about commencing hormone replacment therapy (HRT) and indeed may have relative contraindications. This difficult scenario can be well illustrated by the following case. A 43-year-old woman had developed an early menopause but had had intraductal breast carcinoma 10 years before. Clearly this was a virulent, early onset carcinoma at a very young age and although there was no node involvement she had been treated with axillary clearance, radiotherapy and adjuvant chemotherapy. She had been free of recurrence for the 10-year interval of her follow-up when she came to the menopause clinic with amenorrhoea and profound vasomotor symptoms. There was surprisingly little vaginal dryness but there was diminution in libido (sex drive). Her family history revealed hypertension, late onset diabetes and ischaemic heart disease and her mother had suffered osteoporosis. This woman could appreciate the advantages of HRT: she was fully aware of its cardioprotective effect and her risk of osteoporosis both because of her family history and the fact that she herself had undergone a premature menopause. Nevertheless, she could not bring herself to consider taking HRT in view of her own personal history of breast cancer. Ultimately, when all the facts are given to the woman concerned, the final decision has to be hers.

A number of studies have now suggested that the five-year survival rate following breast cancer is improved in HRT users versus non-users (Bergkvist et al. 1989; Beral 1997).

Contd.

Nonetheless we still lack the definitive evidence obtained from a prospective randomized control trial, and in cases of previous breast cancer the woman's wishes must be paramount. Eventually, after considerable counselling and advice, this particular woman opted for a more holistic approach to healthcare. She is a fit non-smoker who is not overweight and has been advised to pursue weight-bearing exercises in line with the National Osteoporosis Society Guidelines, to take calcium supplementation with a low-fat diet and to consider dietary phytoestrogens. These can be obtained now in Burgen bread and also in red clover capsules from most health food shops. She requires a baseline bone density study, which will need to be repeated in two years' time, and if there is evidence of a fall in bone density bisphosphanates can be considered. She is not a suitable candidate for selective oestrogen receptor modulators (SERMs). Currently, raloxifene is available but can produce sweats and flushes and this woman had experienced quite profound vasomotor symptoms. When the second- and third-generation SERMs are available they may well be able to provide bone and cardiovascular protection without producing side effects or risking stimulation of breast receptors. Norethisterone is also a possible option in that it has a direct effect on bone density in its own right and can be effective in relieving sweats and flushes. The main message to present to this particular woman was that the situation for her was not hopeless. Indeed, if she did not wish to take HRT alternative treatment options were available. She has gone away realizing that a responsible approach to regular surveillance is necessary and that she can elect to opt for some of the other treatment modalities such as norethisterone and biphosphonates.

Haematological malignancies

Ovarian function is invariably affected by the chemotherapeutic regimens employed in the treatment of haematological malignancies (Chatterjee & Goldstone 1996). The degree to which this damage is reversible depends on a number of factors, including age and antecedent treatment. The intensive chemotherapy regimens that accompany bone marrow transplantation often result in permanent gonadal damage (i.e. damage to the reproductive system), although there are an increasing number of reports in the literature documenting recovery of function with spontaneous ovulation. Both total body irradiation and more localized pelvic radiotherapy also result in ovarian damage and, again, the degree to which this is recoverable is dictated by the woman's age, dose of irradiation and previous or concomitant chemotherapy. Transposition procedures to remove ovaries from the treatment field can successfully preserve function.

Women who do not recover gonadal function will often find that, in addition to the known risks of long-term hypo-oestrogenism, they are particularly susceptible to bone loss. As well as the absence of endogenous oestrogen production, both the disease process itself and corticosteroids administered as part of chemotherapy regimens will accelerate the pathophysiological processes leading to osteoporosis. As many of these women will have achieved long-term remission or cure, the complications of osteoporotic bone two or three decades hence are potentially grave. Particular consideration should be given to this when prescribing replacement therapy with use of an androgenic progestogen or, in the event of a contraindication to oestrogen, a biphosphonate.

Fertility issues are a priority in this group of prematurely menopausal women as their diagnosis of malignancy will often have been made prior to them entering the reproductive phase of their lives (see Chapter 9 for discussion of fertility).

Surgical menopause

Women who have undergone premature loss of gonadal function as a result of a surgical menopause must be treated in the context of the underlying disease process that led to this surgery. One indication for which total abdominal hysterectomy and bilateral salpingo-oophorectomy is being increasingly performed is endometriosis. In this circumstance, there is concern that replacement hormonal therapy may lead to a recurrence of the symptoms and signs of the underlying endometriosis. This has therefore given rise to the practice of using combined oestrogen and progestogen replacement, even though the woman no longer requires endometrial protection. We currently use this approach for the first six months of therapy and then continue with single agent oestrogen replacement. Others, though, feel that combined treatment is unnecessary as only a minority of women will experience a relapse following surgery. A further concern of gynaecologists is the timing of HRT in the post-operative period, although recent evidence suggests that immediate treatment is no more likely to cause a recurrence of pain than delayed therapy (Hickman et al. 1998).

Young women who have undergone a surgical menopause often face a rapid decline in libido post-operatively and may benefit from the cautious use of testosterone replacement therapy.

An often forgotten group of women are those who undergo a Wertheim's hysterectomy for Stage 1B or 2A carcinoma of the cervix. Classically, this operation conserves the ovaries as squamous cell carcinoma does not spread to them. However, if the operative specimen demonstrates pelvic nodal involvement, subsequent wide-field radiotherapy will be planned. While these women do not lose ovarian function at the time of surgery, they do lose it with subsequent intervention, by which time oestrogen replacement is sometimes overlooked by the GP and indeed by the specialist oncology unit whose follow-up is aimed at monitoring for recurrence. HRT is not contraindicated in this group of women as the malignancy is not oestrogen-dependent (Gadducci et al. 1997).

It is now commonly accepted practice that women who have undergone surgery for Stage 1, i.e. surgically curative endometrial or ovarian cancer, may have HRT if clear of recurrence for one year.

It is important to remember that women who have hysterectomies with ovarian conservation are likely to experience ovarian failure on average four years earlier than they would otherwise be expected to (Siddle et al. 1987).

Guidelines for good practice in menopause care

Clearly the critical first visit must be handled with care. The woman may be apprehensive, upset and confused; often unable to initially accept that she may be experiencing/has experienced a premature menopause. Others, of course, are only too aware of their predicament since the cessation of ovarian function is secondary to treatment that they have received or surgery that has been performed. In either case, time must be taken to give an adequate amount of information about the condition and the many treatment options available. This is most effectively achieved by providing leaflets, which should be easily comprehensible and, as appropriate, available in a variety of languages depending on the ethnicity of the local population. Videos are another practical way of dispensing information and some general practices now offer a video library, which allows the woman to take the video home and view it with her partner, sharing the information it contains and allowing some discussion to take place in the family circle before returning for further consultation with the clinician (Sethi & Pitkin 1995). Certainly, two or three visits are usually required before the woman is able to decide about long-term treatment. It is not desirable to try to force a decision at the first visit as this may lead to poor adherence long term (Ravnikar 1987). The use of a menopause counsellor in specialized clinics is also advantageous. Counsellors will have more time available to sit and talk through these issues with the woman, particularly in the busy outpatient setting. A practice nurse who has been well-trained may assume this role in a general practice setting.

Once a decision regarding treatment has been made, the first follow-up visit should ideally be three or four months later. It is important to warn the woman of any minor side effects that may occur in the first one or two cycles. These are normally transient and include mastalgia (pain in the breasts) and irregular breakthrough bleeding. Nevertheless, if the woman perseveres, these side effects have normally subsided by the third or fourth cycle. There is therefore little point reviewing the situation prior to this. It is also important to mention that the first withdrawal bleed is usually heavier and possibly more painful then subsequent bleeds and that by the end of the fourth cycle a pattern will emerge.

There is at present much controversy surrounding breast examination. Certainly women should be advised about breast self-awareness. Many general practices feel that they are unable to provide regular breast examination. Practice nurses who often follow up menopausal women do not feel that they are legally covered or have the adequate expertise to perform these examinations. GPs are now reluctant following the Chief Medical Officer's circular (Calman & Moores 1998). Nevertheless, there is certainly an argument, in specialist clinics where personnel are regularly examining breasts, that this practice should continue and indeed it is an opportunity to reinforce the importance of breast self-awareness. Mammography should be performed every five years until the age of 50, when the woman will automatically be eligible for the National Breast Screening Programme offering three-yearly mammography with computer recall. Women with a family history of breast cancer may elect to have more regular screening at 18–24-month intervals. Women under the age of 40 are probably best followed up with breast examination and breast ultrasonography where there is a clinical indication. Bone densitometry should be performed as a baseline where possible, particularly when there is a strong indication, and two- to three-yearly thereafter depending on the response rate observed. The setting for follow-up visits will be dictated largely by the complexity of the clinical situation. Some centres will offer combined clinics on a monthly basis between the specialist menopause clinic and the bone metabolic unit, the breast screening unit or the thrombophilia clinic. These specialist centres may be necessary for women with complex medical problems. For a healthy woman undergoing an idiopathic (unexplained) premature menopause, who appears to be stable and well-controlled on her current hormone replacement regimen, there is no reason why she could not be followed up in the general practice setting.

The cooperation between primary and secondary care is of paramount importance among women who require long-term monitoring, and referral back to a specialist centre may be necessary from time to time if problems ensue. Networking between the local specialist centre and the surrounding general practitioners' surgeries is extremely important, and this can be facilitated through outreach work by nurse specialists, counsellors and even pharmacists (Tanna, 199). The latter are of particular importance when drug interaction issues may be involved. All women experiencing a premature menopause should be provided with a contact number for their local support group, which may be run within the hospital, attached to a local surgery or in the homes of other women with a similar experience. Women should also be given a helpline number whereby they will have access to advice from a specialist nurse or clinician. Ideally, a professional helpline number should be available for GPs or practice nurses who have encountered difficulties so that they can be put in touch with the local specialist centre quickly when necessary.

Adherence

Poor uptake and continuance rates of HRT are of concern in all groups of women for whom it is prescribed, but none more so than for women who experience premature menopause. The prevalence of HRT use has significantly increased in both hysterectomized and non-hysterectomized women under 50 years of age over the past 10 years (Moorhead et al. 1997) but there is little information available about the subgroup of women experiencing premature menopause. It is important that these young women understand the excess metabolic risk at which they are placed by their hypo-oestrogenism and are not treated under the same guidelines as those women who lose ovarian function in the fifth decade of life. Commitment to treatment may be enhanced by ongoing dialogue about the various options, particularly the newer therapeutic alternatives and by open channels of communication as described above.

Ongoing management and follow-up

The predominant controversy with long-term ingestion of HRT is the issue of breast cancer risk. The recent Collaborative Group on Hormonal Factors in Breast Cancer report has attempted to quantify the risk factors based on the length of exposure to oestrogen (Collaborative Group on Hormonal Factors in Breast Cancer 1997). Unfortunately, breast cancer is a common condition with a prevalence of approximately 40 per 1000 women. It is estimated that in women who become menopausal before the age of 50, the risk is decreased consequent to the hypo-oestrogenic state. The prescribing of HRT in this young cohort of women therefore acts to return their risk to that of the general population of women who have maintained their endogenous oestrogen production. The risk does not rise above that of the background female population until after the age of 50 years, when replacement oestrogen is being given at a time when intrinsic production would have ceased. Here it has been estimated that the increased incidence of breast cancer is two additional cases per thousand women after five years of HRT usage, rising to an additional five or six cases after 10 years. One recent study suggests that HRT usage is associated with less aggressive tumour types, when cancer does occur (Gapstur et al. 1999)

The cardioprotective effect of endogenous oestrogen production has been extensively documented in epidemiological studies, with age-matched cohorts who are postmenopausal having a significantly increased risk of cardiovascular disease compared with those who maintain ovarian function. The disparity is even more evident for women who have undergone bilateral oophorectomy. In addition to the prescription of HRT, follow up of a woman's cardiovascular risk assessment includes monitoring blood pressure and lipid profiles, diagnosing and treating diabetes where appropriate, and encouragement not to smoke. Approximately 15–20% of the beneficial effect of HRT on coronary artery disease is derived from its ability to moderate the adverse changes in lipid profiles that accompany the menopause, and some small studies have shown HRT to compare favourably to statins in this regard. Recent British Hyperlipidaemia Association guidelines have endorsed the use of HRT, incorporating a non-androgenic progestogen where there is a requirement for endometrial protection, to treat hyperlipidaemia, suggesting non-oral formulations in cases with elevated triglyceride levels (British Hyperlipidaemia Association 1998).

It is not clear what the optimal length of time for continuing HRT for primary prevention of coronary artery disease is, and the issue has been further complicated by the publication of the US Heart and Estrogen/Progestin Replacement Study (HERS) (Hulley et at. 1998) addressing secondary prevention. This study failed to show a reduction in fatal and non-fatal coronary events, despite the numerous observational studies suggesting an even greater benefit on secondary prevention than that seen with primary prevention (Sullivan et al. 1990). More large prospective studies are needed to clarify these points. At present the reality is that duration of therapy is dictated by the concerns surrounding increasing breast cancer risk after five years.

Follow-up of bone status will depend on the estimated baseline risk. If initial screening confirms early bone loss, osteopaenia or indeed actual osteoporosis, then the woman will require subsequent bone densitometry measurements to assess response to therapy. This may be indicated annually if the osteoporosis is severe, or following 18–24 months of therapy, if the bone loss is not as marked. Five per cent of women are poor responders to this aspect of hormone replacement even when given adequate bone-sparing doses of oestrogen, and this subgroup need to be identified as soon as possible so that alternative or adjuvant therapy with a biphosphonate may be commenced. The role of the new SERMs has yet to be evaluated in this relatively young age group.

Epidemiological studies have suggested that the use of HRT might delay the onset of Alzheimer's dementia and improves certain cognitive modalities in mild cases of already established dementia (Birge 1996). Although the evidence is limited to small studies, it may be of particular relevance to a woman with premature menopause who is potentially facing a prolonged period of hypo-oestrogenism.

Conclusion

The management of women who enter the postmenopausal phase of their lives at a premature age requires a multidisciplinary approach utilizing the skills of menopause specialists, gynaecologists and endocrinologists, and menopause specialist nurses and counsellors. Those women whose loss of ovarian function is as a result of underlying illness or its subsequent treatment will also require input from the relevant specialists. As the number of therapeutic options, both hormonal and non-hormonal, increases and as the range of HRT preparations expands, their place in the therapeutic armamentarium for women with premature menopause needs to be more extensively evaluated.

Chapter 9
Fertility treatments and choices

HOSSAM I ABDALLA AND ANDREW KAN

Introduction

Infertility can be one of the most difficult conseqences of premature menopause for women to deal with. Some women gradually adjust to not having an/other child, while those who want to have children or to have additional children have options, which include fertility treatments and possibly adoption. In this chapter we present up-to-date information about the various fertility treatments available, and some of the moral and ethical issues they raise.

Fertility treatments

Ovum donation

The mainstay of fertility treatment for women with premature menopause is ovum (egg) donation. Other options, such as cryopreservation of ova/ovarian tissue, are still in the experimental stage. Women with premature menopause may be considered ideally suited for ovum donation because better control of the hormonal milieu can be achieved with the absence of functioning hormones and without interference from cyclical ovarian hormones. Once the donated oocytes from volunteers are obtained – and with waiting lists of up to two years this can be a lengthy procedure unless the woman has a willing donor whom she knows – there are several techniques for assisted reproduction. These are in vitro fertilization and embryo transfer (IVF-ET), zygote intrafallopian tube transfer (ZIFT) and gamete intrafallopian tube transfer (GIFT).

Historical background

The use of donated sperm to achieve a pregnancy was first mentioned by Pancoast in 1884 (Finegold 1976). Some 99 years later, after the birth of the first IVF baby was described by Finegold (1976), the first pregnancy using a donated embryo occurred (Trounson et al. 1983). The following year Lutjen and his colleagues (1984) reported the first ongoing pregnancy using IVF of a donated oocyte in a woman with primary ovarian failure (i.e. a woman who had never menstruated). This was followed by the first pregnancies after ZIFT using donated zygotes (Yovich et al. 1987) and GIFT following the transfer of donated oocytes (Asch et al. 1988). The application of cryopreservation followed later that same year when Abdalla and Leonard reported the first successful birth following ZIFT of a cryopreserved zygote derived from a donated oocyte (Abdalla & Leonard 1988).

Assessment

When a woman with premature menopause is referred for infertility treatment, it is important to assess both the woman and her partner, to confirm the diagnosis and elucidate a cause for the premature menopause by means of history, examination and investigation. Pelvic ultrasound and/or hysteroscopy may be required to ascertain whether there is abnormality of the uterus. Semen analysis should be done to exclude any additional male factor as a cause of infertility. In the event of a low sperm count or other abnormality, intracytoplasmic sperm injection (ICSI) may be considered; where there is no sperm even with sperm retrieval, donor sperm may be needed.

Egg collection

The donor is given hormonal drugs to stimulate her ovaries in order to mature several oocytes in one monthly cycle. Follicular development is monitored by ultrasonic measurements and/or serum oestradiol levels. Human chorionic gonadotrophin (hCG) is given to mature the oocytes 34–38 hours before retrieval under either local or general anaesthesia. Retrieval is carried out on a day-care basis, under either local or general anaesthesia. The oocytes are usually collected through the vagina with the aid of transvaginal ultrasonography.

Semen collection

On the day of oocyte retrieval, the male partner is asked to produce a semen sample. The sample is prepared and the oocyte insemi-nated. If donor sperm is used, the sample is taken from frozen stor-age and prepared for insemination.

Synchronization

In a natural cycle, embryonic and endometrial development is dependent on the cyclical production of ovarian hormones, whereas in an egg donation cycle ovarian stimulation of the donor and endometrial preparation of the recipient are separate events which need to be coordinated. While the donor is undergoing ovarian stim-ulation in preparation for egg collection, the recipient must undergo hormonal treatment to prepare the uterus for implantation of the embryo. Endometrial development appears to be the critical factor in assessment of the efficacy of various regimens of hormone replacement therapy (HRT). The effective oral dose of oestradiol seems to be between 2 and 8 mg per day, while the effective proges-terone dose lies between 25 and 100 mg per day administered by intramuscular injection or 300 mg a day per vaginum. The success-ful use of fixed doses of steroids, as compared to earlier use of incre-mental doses, has improved and simplified protocols (Younis et al. 1996). As there are individual variations in response to therapy, a pre-treatment 'dummy cycle' to evaluate histological and endocrino-logical responses is recommended (Sauer et al. 1997).

IVF-ET

Once the oocytes and semen have been collected and prepared, they are placed together in a dish in an incubator. The dish is inspected the following day to see whether fertilization has occurred. If the oocytes have been fertilized, the resulting embryos are left to divide for between two and five days. The embryologist checks that the embryos are developing normally and up to three embryos (depend-ing on the IVF unit) are transferred into the recipient's uterus via the cervix. A pregnancy test is performed two weeks later to determine whether treatment has been successful.

GIFT

GIFT is a technique in which oocytes and prepared semen are trans-ferred to one or both fallopian tubes, usually by means of laparo-scopically directed tubal cannulation. Fertilization occurs in vivo.

The first successful pregnancy following GIFT was reported in 1984 by Asch and colleagues. After the donor oocytes and the partner's sperm have been collected, a laparoscopy is performed. The partner's prepared semen, together with an agreed number of oocytes separated by a bubble in the transfer catheter, are gently discharged into the preampullary area of the fallopian tube. The result of this union is unknown because the development of zygotes cannot be seen. Consequently IVF is often performed at the same time as GIFT, to provide an indication of the likely outcome of the eggs and semen transferred to the fallopian tube. Resulting embryos can be frozen for possible future use.

Advantages of GIFT include in vivo fertilization, and less specialized equipment and fewer trained personnel than are required for IVF. Disadvantages of GIFT include the loss of information regarding fertilization (unless IVF with excess oocytes or pregnancy results), and the risk of general anaesthesia and surgery associated with laparoscopy. GIFT is contraindicated when there is significant tubal damage or pelvic adhesions.

ZIFT

ZIFT is the laparoscopic transfer of zygote(s) into the fallopian tube after oocyte fertilization in vitro. We include under ZIFT other procedures known as tubal embryo transfer (TET) and pronuclear stage transfer (PROST). These procedures differ only in the stage of development at which the embryos are transferred: in PROST the pronuclear stage, in ZIFT the two-cell stage and in TET beyond the two-cell stage.

The ZIFT protocol entails ovarian stimulation and oocyte collection, IVF of oocytes and then laparoscopic or transcervical tubal embryo transfer. Highlighted in this protocol is the need for IVF and embryo transfer to the fallopian tube, which is performed one to three days after fertilization. The advantages are confirmation of fertilization and transfer of the embryo to the optimal site, i.e. the fallopian tube, where the environment is more conducive to the developing embryo than is the uterine cavity.

Embryo donation

A further medical treatment available to women with premature menopause is embryo donation. Donation of excess embryos from

IVF treatment to the woman of an infertile couple has long been possible but the practice is not widespread because it poses ethical, legal and psychological dilemmas.

There are two ways to proceed with embryo donation. One way would be to obtain separate egg and sperm donation; the resultant embryos, after fertilization, are then placed in the recipient's uterus. In this case the embryos are created from two separate gamete donations, most likely from two persons unknown to each other. A second way is to obtain embryos produced by another couple in their attempts at pregnancy through IVF but which they no longer need or want.

The degree to which embryo donation is successful will depend primarily on the viability of donated embryos. If donated embryos are created from separate egg and sperm donations, the success rate should approach that of egg donation. This is higher than basic IVF because most donor eggs come from younger healthier women. A 30% take-home baby rate per retrieval cycle may be expected from embryos freshly created from separate sperm and egg donations (American Fertility Society 1994). The success rate for donations of excess or unwanted embryos is likely to be considerably less. Excess embryos not previously chosen for transfer may be of poorer quality; and they may also be from older women whose oocytes are generally not as good as those of younger women.

Success rate of ovum donation

In general, most egg donor programmes have achieved a higher pregnancy rate than those found in regular IVF treatment (Sauer 1996), although it remains unclear whether this difference is a result of endometrial receptivity or oocyte quality or a combination of both. Several studies have been conducted in this area but results are not yet conclusive. Davies et al. (1990) suggested endometrial receptivity is a key factor in conception while Schwartz et al. (1997) concluded that embryo quality was the most reliable predictor of pregnancy outcome.

It is known that fertility in women declines with age (Rosenwaks et al. 1995); strikingly so after 35 years (Yovich et al. 1987), and is all but lost by the age of 45 (Asch et al. 1988). To establish whether this age-related reproductive failure might result from either a problem in the uterus/endometrium or poor oocyte quality, Sauer et al.

(1990) compared the outcome of oocyte donation among women aged 40 to 44 years and those under 40 years. They described eight embryo transfers which resulted in five viable pregnancies, one with twins. A sixth pregnancy ended in miscarriage. Five normal infants were delivered vaginally. They compared the outcome with those of women under 40 with ovarian failure who also had oocyte donation and with ovulating women 40 or older who were undergoing standard IVF. Sauer and his team found no significant difference in the rate of implantation or ongoing pregnancy between older and younger women receiving oocyte donation. These rates were significantly higher than in the infertile ovulating women of a similar age undergoing standard IVF treatment. The authors concluded that the endometrium retains its ability to respond to gonadal steroids and provides a receptive environment for embryo implantation and gestation regardless of age.

In a much larger study, Abdalla et al. (1990) initially reported a decline in pregnancy rates with age as pregnancy was achieved in only 9% of women over 40, despite the fact that the age of the donor was not significantly different between the two groups. However, this decline in the pregnancy rate was no longer true when they analysed the results of their first three years' experience (371 cycles) of oocyte donation (7th World Congress, unpublished data). In a more recent study, the same group of investigators published a study in which they matched every recipient aged 39 years or less with a recipient aged between 40 and 52, with a minimum of five years difference (Abdalla et al. 1997). Matched recipients received oocytes from the same donor and a total of 52 transfer cycles was performed in each age group (young versus old). There were no differences in pregnancy (38.5% versus 38.5%), delivery (25% versus 23%) and miscarriage rates (35% versus 40%). This finding was supported by a study by Paulson et al. (1997), who found that age and endometrial receptivity were unrelated. In contrast Borini et al. (1996) reported that pregnancy and implantation rates were higher in women under 40 compared to those over 40 and concluded that this difference was due to uterine factors. Their study showed no significant difference in the miscarriage rate between the two groups. Table 9.1 is a summary of studies that have been performed to resolve this vexed question of whether the success of oocyte donation is related to the age of the recipient. On balance of evidence it would appear that the age of recipient does not have as much of an influence on ovum

Table 9.1: Pregnancy per cycle related to age of recipient*

	Group A (age < =39 years)	Group B (age >= 40 years)
Navot et al. 1994 (49)	11/51 (21.5%)	12/51 (23.5%)
Cano et al. 1995 (50)	21/45 (46.7%)	25/45 (55.5%)
Borini et al. 1996 (33)	27/57 (47.8%)	14/57 (24.5%)
Abdalla et al. 1997 (31)	20/52 (38.5%)	20/52 (38.5%)
Total	79/205 (38.5%)	71/205* (34.6%)

*$\chi^2 = 0.513$, DF = 1, P = 0.473 NS

donation cycles as compared to assisted conceptions cycles using one's own eggs.

Risk

The recipient following a successful oocyte donation cycle is in a unique position of carrying a fetus to whom she has not contributed any genetic material. Whether she is at increased obstetric risk, apart from other confounding factors such as age or multiple pregnancy, has been the subject of a number of reports (Pados et al. 1994; Sauer et al. 1995; Soderstrom-Antilla & Hovatta 1995). Abdalla et al. (1998) confirmed the finding of Pados and colleagues (1994) of an increased incidence of pregnancy-induced hypertension in recipients of ovum donation. Pados et al. had found an incidence of 23% in 232 oocyte donation pregnancies compared with Abdalla's one third (33%). Other findings of Abdalla and colleagues include a high (11%) incidence of postpartum haemorrhage, with 6% requiring a blood transfusion, and an increased incidence of small-for-gestational-age babies, especially in women with ovarian failure. These women were also found to have a significantly higher incidence of miscarriage compared with those with functioning ovaries. Although the overall pregnancy rate was higher than among those with functioning ovaries, the rate of successful pregnancy was not significantly different because of the increased incidence of early pregnancy loss (miscarriage) in women with ovarian failure. It seems prudent therefore that such women should be under the care of a consultant obstetrician, and cross-matched blood should be available throughout pregnancy and especially in the period just after delivery.

Moral and ethical issues

As treatment options proliferate and become more accessible, moral and ethical concerns regarding the physical and emotional health of all parties involved have been raised. These are usually discussed in terms of three philosophical principles: autonomy, beneficence and justice. The principle of autonomy implies that human beings are not commodities and have the right to accurate information about themselves to give informed consent. Beneficence refers to doing good to others but becomes problematic where the risks and benefits of treatment are not clear-cut. Justice usually refers to the fair distribution of the benefits and burdens of treatment in a population. However, in relation to infertility and its treatment, along with notions of 'family', the issues are extremely complex and psychological dilemmas become intertwined with ethical ones.

One of the most difficult issues surrounding oocyte donation is the question of who is the mother of the child conceived from oocyte donation. The biological/genetic mother may not be the same person as the 'carrying' (or gestational) mother and neither need be the social mother. Most people (including the law in the UK) usually consider the mother to be the woman who gives birth to the child.

Others, for example couples undergoing surrogacy, may have a different view. The definition of motherhood often depends on the particular fertility predicament. To the couple pursuing surrogacy, the genetic source of the oocytes is often the single most important factor. On the other hand, couples receiving donor oocytes may be more likely to consider the mother who gives birth to the child as the 'real' mother. Notions of what constitutes a 'real' mother have been extended by the advent of fertility treatments. A woman can be the biological parent, non-biological social parent or an egg donor. She may be fertile or infertile, single or married, heterosexual or homosexual. Similarly the idea of fatherhood, always perhaps precarious in the past, has become an even more relative concept. A man too can be a biological parent, non-biological social parent or a sperm donor. Like the woman, he may be fertile, infertile, single, married, heterosexual or homosexual, or a combination of the above.

SURROGACY

In 1996 a joint Human Fertilisation and Embryology Authority (HFEA) and British Medical Association (BMA) leaflet distinguished between two types of surrogacy: in 'partial' surrogacy (also known as traditional or straight surrogacy) the surrogate mother provides the egg; and the sperm from the intended father is placed into the surrogate mother, either by the surrogate herself (self-insemination) or by a health professional at a clinic. From then on fertilization occurs in the usual way. With full (also known as host or IVF surrogacy) the surrogate mother has no genetic link with the child but gestates embryos usually created from the egg and sperm of the intended (social) parents. The procedure involves collecting the eggs from the intended mother and sperm from the intended father, and placing them together in the laboratory. One or more (a maximum of three, usually two) embryos are placed into the surrogate's uterus for gestation. Where the intended mother cannot produce eggs herself, as in premature menopause, an embryo can be created from the sperm of the intended father and eggs from an anonymous (or known) donor, also using IVF techniques. Similarly, if the intended father is infertile, donor sperm can be used.

Opposition to surrogate parenting, particularly those that involve monetary exchange, has been made on moral grounds as third-party baby-selling (Salzer 1991) and fears of it leading to an 'underclass of breeder women' (Holbrook 1990). Supporters of the practice justify financial recognition of the time, effort and pain of bearing the child, although most of the women who undertake surrogacy cite altruistic reasons (for a personal account of surrogacy in the UK, see Cotton 1992). Often the emphasis is on parental rights, obligations and responsibilities (Parker 1984). Certainly less is known of the children's views. Ethically a balance needs to be found between the wishes of the intended parents and the

Contd.

autonomy and wellbeing of the surrogate mother while she is carrying a child (Jaeger 1996), and the psychological well-being of the future child. Currently in the UK, surrogacy arrangements are not illegal but payment of surrogate mothers, even of expenses, is increasingly discouraged.

While many women anxious to achieve pregnancy are favourably disposed towards egg donation, the degree of social support that they will receive depends in part on attitudes in the wider social environment. A survey of public opinion showed that more than half of the responders of both sexes were favourably disposed towards egg donation. Men exhibited significantly more positive attitudes towards oocyte donation by a partner's sister than did women (Lessor et al. 1991). In theory the donation of oocytes should parallel the donation of semen, but there are important differences. Oocyte donation inevitably requires the donor to undergo the inconvenience accompanied by the potential hazards of ovarian hyperstimulation and oocyte recovery (Bromwich 1990). In addition, where the egg donor is known, or is a member of the family, the question of whether the donor may feel she has the right to intervene in the family dynamics or with the child could arise.

Another important issue is that of disclosure: whether the rearing or social parents should tell the child of his or her genetic origin. From a psychological point of view it has been argued that secrets can have a detrimental effect on the family unit by placing a deception at the centre of the most basic human relationships. So far the parents of children born using assisted reproductive technology have received inconsistent messages from health professionals regarding the implications of openness as against secrecy and little research has as yet been published in this area.

A comparison with adoption has frequently been made in relation to the conflict between the child's right to know and the parents' right to privacy (for the experience of adoptees see Triseliotis 1973; Harper 1993). The similarity between the issues faced by adoptees and those of offspring of donor gametes remains a subject of debate (Cook et al. 1995). Arguably, families created through the use of donated gametes are families 'with a difference' – a difference that may need to be valued rather than rendered negative by making it to conform to something it is not (McDonald 1997). This point is reiterated by Daniels (1997), who emphasizes that openness and information-sharing make for strong, healthy family relationships, built on trust and honesty and so better able to withstand fluctuating family circumstances.

Openness has been actively promoted by social workers working with adoption since the legal rights of adoptees to know their origins was enacted in 1975 in the UK. This is viewed as a way to establish the 'the normality of telling', whereas lack of disclosure may imply concealment of something shameful or unpleasant and act as a potential for harm, which is greater the longer the information is kept secret. Telling itself is increasingly viewed as an ongoing process, different aspects of which figure more or less prominently according to the development of the individual and the family unit (Blyth 1998).

The need for donor anonymity is certainly complex. While some donor offspring and some recipient parents may press for the 'right to know', donors themselves may be reluctant to have contact with offspring engendered in this way, and other recipient couples may feel apprehensive and confused about a child's feelings towards his or her (genetic/social) identity. The UK regulatory body, the Human Fertilisation and Embryology Authority (HFEA), has guidelines which allow certain information about donors to be known to the recipient, but this remains a controversial area. Kirkland and colleagues (1992) found that 63% of donors would still donate if the recipient was given their name, but only 23% of recipients would agree to receive oocytes if their name was made available to the donor. Similarly 70% of donors preferred to donate to someone they knew, whereas only 44% of recipients were willing to accept eggs from a known donor. Although more than half (55%) of donors did not object to being contacted when the children were adults, an overwhelming 90% of recipients were opposed to the idea. Generally, but to different degrees, both donors (71%) and recipients (86%) preferred anonymity. Although 86% of donors wanted to know the outcome of their donations, 80% denied any desire for a connection with that child. Thus there appeared to be a consensus among donors and recipients that gestational parentage is more significant than genetic parentage.

In a smaller survey in Canada, anonymity was found to be a primary concern for both recipients and donors, with 80% of couples not planning to inform the child of his or her origin (Khamsi et al. 1997). In the few studies which have been carried out in the UK, disclosure remains uncommon, despite the belief of counsellors and social workers that openness is the best policy (McWhinnie 1996). Much of the above research has been carried out with semen donation; more research is needed to clarify attitudes and beliefs about egg donation.

Health implications are also involved in the issue of disclosure. The increased emphasis on the importance of genetic inheritance for health and life span has prompted concern among some parents of donor offspring, particularly those of donor sperm, about the possibility of being carriers of a defective gene and the risk of consanguinity. However small the chances, some believe there is the possibility of committing 'accidental incest' with a half sibling or of their children marrying a first cousin, with possible implications for genetic abnormalities as well as the social stigma associated with incest (Daniels 1997; Lauren 1998; Whipp 1998). This has been taken into account by HFEA guidelines, which allow for the provision of information as to the relationship between two people who wish to marry, where one or both were born as a result of gamete donation. A related issue is the possibility of analysing the genetic material of donor gametes or embryos, which could influence selection of donors. On the positive side this could avoid the implantation of gametes that carry certain genetic disorders but it also raises fears of creating a 'super race' (Cooper-Hilbert 1998).

The 1998 HFEA Code of Practice in the UK stresses the importance of considering the welfare of the potential child by stating that fertility clinics should take into account:

> a child's potential need to know about their origins and whether or not the prospective parents are prepared for the questions which may arise while the child is growing up.

However, at the time of writing, under legislation enacted in 1990, donor offspring are legally able to access only the most basic information regarding their donor. This consists of non-identifying information, primarily physical characteristics, which are made available either when the child reaches the age of majority – 18 years or earlier (usually 16 years) in special circumstances, such as when the information is relevant to an impending marriage.

HFEA GUIDELINES

The HFEA produces a number of leaflets which outline the legal position of egg donors and what they might expect in terms of treatment, responsibilities and rewards (see Resources). It keeps a register of names and the age of donors. Egg donors are advised that, although they are a genetic parent, they have no claim on the child under the law and equally no responsibilities. The donor's name is kept on a confidential register. The only exception occurs when a child is born with a disability as a result of the donor's failure to disclose inherited disease so that these children can seek legal redress in the courts. Additional information that is currently collected but not divulged may be made available to the child as an adult through some future act of Parliament, but under the 1990 Act names cannot be divulged retrospectively.

It is a statutory obligation of all clinics to have counselling available for anyone undergoing fertility treatment. The HFEA outlines three types of counselling which may help during treatment. The first is implications counselling, which must be made available to everyone and deals with the implications of treatment both for the couple and for the resulting child. The second is support counselling. This aims to offer emotional help at particularly stressful times before, during or after treatment. Third is therapeutic counselling, which concerns itself with the wider aspects of infertility and treatment. This third form of counselling may be provided by specialists outside the clinic.

HFEA leaflets
- Becoming an Egg or Sperm Donor
- In Vitro Fertilisation (IVF Treatment)
- Choosing a Fertility Treatment Centre
- The HFEA Code of Practice

In the US, conception is largely unregulated: the right to privacy is enshrined in the constitution, effectively protecting reproductive decisions and granting couples autonomy regardless of other concerns, such as suitability as parents. Those who favour disclosure have argued that a commitment to openness can only be of value if it is backed by the force of legal obligation.

Internationally the picture varies from country to country. In Victoria, Australia, the Infertility Treatment Act 1995 came into force on 1 January 1998. It stipulates that any person donating gametes is potentially identifiable to the offspring created when they reach 18 years of age, as well as to donors, to parents of donor offspring/recipients of donated gametes and to descendants of donor offspring. In the past the fear has been expressed that the availability of identifying information will end the availability of donor gametes. Certainly at present a shortage of egg donors persists.

This raises another important ethical question as to whether there should be monetary reward to, in particular, egg donors (Balen & Jacobs 1997; Craft et al. 1997). Across countries, positions vary according to the predominant social value, egalitarianism (equal access to treatment) or libertarianism (treatment if you can afford it), or where a regulatory or facilitative approach predominates. France and New Zealand adopt the view that donations are genuine altruistic gifts requiring no form of compensation. In the UK, payments to egg donors are considered unethical but expenses can be reimbursed to the donor. It can be argued that no money should be paid for embryo donations because of the appearance it gives of putting a financial price on human life. In addition, payments might induce couples to donate embryos they otherwise would have discarded, left in storage or used themselves. In the USA, there is a 'free market' economy in this respect, with access to donors over the Internet. Those who can afford it may opt for treatment in the USA or elsewhere – a phenomenon dubbed 'procreative tourism', which in itself carries a number of potential ethical and moral pitfalls (Nielson 1996).

Part of the difficulty with ovum donation specifically is the highly controversial area of the degree of risk of ovarian cancer from ovarian hyperstimulation. The risk appears to be small but significant and raises a troublesome ethical issue since the donor receives no tangible benefit. Overall, however, there is a slight move towards more openness and access to information in oocyte donation. Kirkland et al. (1992) found that women recipients of oocyte donation were equally divided with regard to the question of telling the child. Power and her colleagues (1990) reported that two-thirds of donors thought they would not want to know of their genetic origin had they been born using a donated egg. Similarly Bertrand-Servais et al. (1993) suggested that donor anonymity allowed oocyte recipients to impose their own identity patterns on to the future child and to introduce him or her in an unbiased way to their own lives. Robertson (1989) noted that the separation of female genetic material and parenting that occurs in egg donation appears to pose the least risk of family conflict or psychological confusion for the offspring.

Embryo donation involves no additional manipulation of embryos beyond those involved in IVF, even if separate gamete donations are used to create the donated embryos. The unique feature of embryo donation is that a child will be born to a couple with whom he or she has no parental genetic tie. In this respect, embryo donation differs from most other methods of assisted reproduction, which involve one or both rearing parents being a genetic parent. The child also differs from adopted children because adopted children have already been born before rearing parents are sought. In sperm donation, the rearing mother provides the egg and gestates; in egg donation the gestational and rearing mother will not be the genetic mother, but the rearing male will be the genetic father. In the case of full surrogacy, the rearing woman will have no biological connection with the child but the rearing man will be the genetic father.

Robertson (1989) argued that this unique feature should not make embryo donation ethically more problematic, especially when children born to embryo donation are compared to those born using other donor or surrogate techniques. In either case, the child resulting from embryo donation would be born to loving parents who have committed themselves to its birth before implantation. Such a child may be much less likely to feel the rejection or abandonment that can be a salient issue for some adopted children. Robertson went on to stress the importance of informed consent and counselling for both donors and recipients in order to consider and minimize the ethical risks. He suggested that all the risks and uncertainties in the procedure of embryo donation should be fully disclosed to both parties. For donors this will include informing them of the social, psychological and legal uncertainties of donation; the risks that a birth may not occur; and the fact that in many clinics they will probably not have any knowledge of or contact with a child who is their genetic offspring. Donors should also be offered implications counselling and should not be used as donors if they have not adequately worked through these issues. (For a further discussion of ethical implications of embryo donation see Warnock 1998.)

Equally, recipients need to be fully informed about the likelihood of pregnancy and birth not occurring; the extent to which genetic and infectious disease screening tests have been done; the risks of disease in the few cases in which screening has not occurred; the psychological uncertainties involved in this parenting arrangement; the extent to which the donors will be informed of their identity and the child's birth; and legal uncertainties about parentage. Recipients should also be offered implications counselling and screened to ensure that they are prepared psychologically to handle the rearing of a genetically unrelated child. In addition, they should be advised on the issues of disclosure and how the child might be helped to deal with information at different stages of his or her development.

The question of disclosure versus maintaining secrecy of origins is an unresolved issue in assisted reproduction. Implications counselling is extremely important; the couple need to be asked to consider the advantages of disclosure and openness, and be enabled to make a decision based on the best interests of the welfare of the child. If disclosure does occur, the child may eventually wish to have information concerning his or her genetic parents.

In short, embryo donation is one way of treating women with premature menopause, but how big a role it will play is not yet clear. When embryo donation is performed, it is important that it be carried out in a manner respectful of all parties. This means full disclosure of medical, social and legal risks and consideration of the psychological implications for donors, recipients and offspring. Legal pitfalls such as the possibility of future custody battles over cryopreserved embryos also need to be considered, as was seen in the US court case (Davis v Davis 1989), as do potential pitfalls such as whether a couple could sue if they did not achieve pregnancy with their own embryos when another couple was successful (Crockin 1997). However, with careful attention to the issues discussed, embryo donation may be practised in an ethically and legally sound way that is mutually satisfying for all parties.

Cryopreservation of human oocytes or ovarian tissue

The possibility of premature menopause and ensuing infertility becomes a very real concern for women who are about to receive chemotherapy or radiotherapy, or undergo a surgical procedure. Although cryopreservation of human embryos has been possible since 1983 (Trounson & Mohr 1983), cryopreservation of ova/ovarian tissue is still not a viable option. To date only five, live-born infants have been reported from untold numbers of attempts to freeze-store oocytes (Oktay et al. 1988). Results have been especially poor following cryopreservation of mature or immature oocytes. Better results followed ovarian tissue-banking, especially in mice (Parrot 1960) and sheep (Gosden et al. 1994). Although ovarian tissue has been successfully frozen and thawed, there has been only one attempt to graft tissue back in humans (Gosden, 1999) and the moral status of the pre-embryo remains highly controversial (Balen & Jacobs 1997).

Alternatives to biological parenting

Adoption

In the present climate, adoption is often considered a 'second-best' choice by the majority of infertile couples (Miall 1987; Sandlowski et al. 1989). This raises the question as to the extent to which our culture emphasizes genetic ties over emotional attachments (Bartholet 1993). In the UK, factors that deter many couples from this option include cumbersome, psychologically intrusive procedures aimed at judging who makes a suitable parent – an arduous process that most other parents do not have to undergo. The degree to which fertility clinics ought to act as 'gatekeepers' in this respect remains highly debated (Leiblum 1997). When considering adoption, couples often worry that the child may have special needs and exhibit unacceptable or deviant behaviour. If the child is from a Third World country, cultural differences may be considered an additional adjustment which may be particularly hard to make while mourning loss of fertility. Some couples reject adoption because the child is neither genetically nor gestationally theirs (Van Balen et al. 1997). Most importantly perhaps from the point of view of the would-be parents, the child may be just that, already a child, rather than a newborn.

There are few babies available for adoption, with the possible exception of overseas adoption. In the UK, couples are required to abandon fertility treatment as soon as they decide to proceed with adoption on the grounds that if they were to conceive the adopted child might be made to feel less welcome. This is not a requirement in the USA. In the UK, the process of being accepted as an adoptive couple can take anywhere between nine months and two years, sometimes longer. Adoption is not usually an option for women without a heterosexual partner. (For an exposition on adoption in the UK see Brodzinsky and Schecter 1990; Howe 1998; in the USA, see Chapter 7, Deveraux & Hammerman 1998.)

Fostering

Fostering tends not to be a satisfactory option for couples who want to have a child or create a family of their own, as the fostered child is not legally theirs. The child may be removed by agencies and returned to the biological parents or other caretakers at any time. In addition, the foster child is often perceived as having a problematic background and expected to show difficult behaviour. As with adoption, the feeling that the foster child is genetically unrelated may be considered a drawback for potential foster parents.

Deciding to not have a child

An insidious aspect of infertility is its tendency to overwhelm all other aspects of life. It can be hard to think of life without children as a positive choice rather than as remaining stuck in a negative state of 'childlessness'. This decision is not made easier in the face of cultural expectations to reproduce; and it is often hard for couples to accept themselves and be understood as well-adjusted, complete families fulfilling other aspects of adulthood such as pursuing lifelong ambitions of world travel and artistic endeavours. It can be overlooked that not having a child does not mean no involvement with children.

Some women with premature menopause may have already had children but have to face the closure of future choices. Others might not have planned to have children. Adjustment to the lack of choice and to not having their own (genetic) children is usually a painful process that many women with premature menopause have to confront. Van Balen et al. (1997) surveyed 131 infertile couples. The authors found that 8% had chosen to remain child-free and pursue other life goals and that this option tended to be chosen late in the course of treatment. Such couples argued that children did not constitute the only thing that made life meaningful; that medical opportunities had been exhausted and that 'you have to do something'. For them, talent and career successes could be valued again after their self-esteem had been battered by the failure to conceive. For men and women who decide not to have a child or not to have any more children, new meanings may be found both spiritually and practically, for example, in helping others with similar problems or by moving into different creative endeavours.

The future

There are two critical areas in the research of fertility treatment for women with premature menopause. If we as medical practitioners could devise a method of reliably predicting which women will have premature menopause and have the facility to cryopreserve ova/ovarian tissue, we would have solved many of the problems associated with premature menopause and fertility.

There is a small group of women whose premature menopause is iatrogenically induced. These include women undergoing chemotherapy and/or radiotherapy for malignancies, such as carcinoma of the breast or leukaemia, and women who have had bilateral oophorectomies. We can predict when these women will be menopausal. However, the majority of women with premature ovarian failure do not have an identifiable etiology. A family history of a mother or a close relative having premature menopause may be significant, but there may be no other indication of premature menopause. The challenge for the future is to devise a screening test to predict which women are at risk of premature ovarian dysfunction so that they could be offered the option of preserving ovarian tissue or oocytes for future use. Traditionally the way to test for ovarian reserve has been a baseline (day 2 to day 5) follicle-stimulating hormone (FSH) and luteinizing hormone (LH) in a natural cycle. Unfortunately this method is neither reliable nor reproducible. Numerous other alternatives have been proposed (including the G test, inhibin, clomid challenge test), but they are no better than the baseline FSH and LH and are often more expensive and time-consuming.

In January 2000 the UK Human Fertilisation and Embryology Authority (HFEA) agreed to lift an earlier ban on the use of frozen oocytes/eggs. This means that women can now store their own frozen, health eggs for future use.

Embryo cryopreservation has become well-established since its introduction in 1983. This technology can be used for women in whom ovarian failure is predicted; ovaries can be hyperstimulated, oocytes collected and fertilized with the partner's sperm, and the resulting embryos cyropreserved. This presupposes that the women have partners at the time and so is unlikely to be appropriate for young persons. The ideal would be to cryopreserve oocytes or ovarian tissue which would also solve the problems of synchronization and markedly reduce the need for oocyte donors.

In conclusion, there are a variety of fertility treatments available to women with a premature menopause who wish to pursue the goal of having children. At present, success rates are modest, with ovum donation appearing to be the best option, but finding a suitable donor can prove difficult.

Chapter 10
Complementary medicine and non-medical approaches

JANET BROCKIE

Whether their menopause is 'on time' or early, some women experience menopausal symptoms that will affect their quality of life and for which they will seek treatment. Increasing numbers of women seek relief of these symptoms from non-conventional therapies and through lifestyle and dietary changes, rather than opting for pharmacological treatments.

Those women who do seek treatment from their GPs most frequently present with uncomfortable menopausal symptoms such as hot flushes and night sweats. Studies have shown that knowledge about the long-term effects of the menopause is generally poor. However, young women who have experienced a premature menopause are more at risk of long-term health problems, such as cardiovascular disease and osteoporosis, and it is essential to consider long-term health as well as short-term discomfort from menopausal symptoms. There are non-medical treatments and complementary therapies available for menopausal symptoms and for the long-term metabolic effects of the menopause that can provide realistic alternatives to conventional medicine.

Conventional medicine primarily offers the menopausal woman hormone replacement therapy (HRT), and a single preparation containing oestrogen can effectively reverse all the effects caused by the decline of oestrogen production by the ovaries at the menopause. Other pharmacological alternatives are available for the control of menopausal symptoms and for the prevention of bone loss. However, some women are choosing to avoid medical solutions and seek help from non-conventional and non-medical approaches, which consist of treatments generally not provided by orthodox healthcare professionals. The reasons for declining mainstream medicine are varied and individual, influenced by medical history and previous experience of healthcare.

Both conventional and non-conventional medicine have their place in healthcare. For life-threatening conditions, surgery and powerful drugs are essential. The term complementary therapies is used in this chapter because it is recognized that there may be times when it is necessary to use orthodox, conventional medicine alongside non-conventional therapies, the two complementing each other, and times when complementary and alternative approaches are used instead of orthodox medicine.

The approaches considered in this chapter include the role of complementary therapies and dietary and lifestyle changes. The role of support groups is considered in Chapter 11.

Why do women want to try complementary and non-medical approaches?

Despite the wealth of medical literature showing the beneficial effects of HRT, only about 17% of women aged between 45 and 69 years elect to take HRT and only a small number continue therapy to maximize the long-term effects of therapy (Hope et al. 1998). The reasons why women elect not to take HRT or to continue to take it are numerous and complex.

For a number of women HRT is contraindicated. Most frequently this is due to a history of oestrogen-dependent carcinoma, usually of the breast or endometrium. Many young women will have experienced a premature menopause as a result of treatment of their disease with radiotherapy or chemotherapy and may experience devastating symptoms made worse by continued treatment of the disease. Other contraindications include chronic active liver disease and a history of venous thromboembolism.

Although there has been much medical research evaluating the effects of HRT, little has specifically looked at the effect of long-term use in young women and this is of concern particularly in relation to breast cancer (Willis et al. 1996). Fear of breast cancer is probably the single most significant obstacle limiting the acceptance of HRT. Other women believe that the menopause is a natural event in a woman's life and should not be interfered with. Some women are concerned about the side effects of HRT, many are convinced that HRT induces obesity (although scientific evidence does not support this). The continuation of vaginal bleeding can be a disincentive, although with newer preparations and treatment regimens, period-free HRT is now available for more women (Okon et al. 1997).

Some women may seek alternative treatments because of a disappointing experience with HRT, while others choose complementary therapies alongside orthodox treatments in a supporting role, helping the body and the mind to develop greater resilience. Lifestyle and dietary changes aimed at promoting good long-term health need to be encouraged at all times and with all age groups. A premature menopause, although distressing, can be an opportunity for women to reassess life plans. For others there is a desire to be more in control of their own treatment. Non-medical alternatives and complementary therapies can allow people to take a greater role in the decisions about treatment and to be more actively involved in promoting good long-term health.

Cross-cultural experiences of the menopause

Cross-cultural research suggests that the meanings attached to the menopause are socially constructed and the way in which the menopause is perceived and experienced is influenced by the status and role of women within a particular society.

The age of the menopause is fairly consistent worldwide, around the age of 50 years. However, the severity and reporting of menopausal symptoms varies enormously. Differences may also be due to a number of other factors, such as genetics, diet, exercise, education, smoking, the environment, attitudes and beliefs. In Asian cultures fewer symptoms are experienced; in Japan, the prevalence of hot flushes is approximately 20% (Lock 1991) – about 80% of women in the UK experience flushes or sweats.

Studies examining cultural differences are difficult to undertake and interpret. Do some cultures reporting a low incidence of flushes do so because in that culture there is no word to express how the woman feels? Or do women in some cultures complain of fewer flushes because their diets reduce symptomatology or because they are embarrassed? Perhaps their society places a high value on stoicism or the menopause is a natural phenomenon that brings certain privileges. Among Rajput women in India, the menopause enables women who have been previously veiled and secluded in purdah to come out from women's quarters to talk and drink with the men (Flint 1975).

Despite these confusing factors, the menopause seems to be associated with fewer and less severe symptoms in Asia than in Western countries. A study looking at the menopause in seven Asian countries reported that the menopause does not assume the importance in the East that it seems to in the West (McCarthy 1990).

There are perhaps lessons to learn from other cultures and their attitude towards the menopause, which differs enormously to the Western cultures. Moreover, within British culture, Hunter (1992) found that women with negative stereotyped beliefs before the menopause are more likely to experience emotional reactions when they reach the menopause.

Non-medical alternatives and complementary therapies allow women themselves to take control of their treatment and play an active role in decision making about their long-term future health, whereas pharmacological treatment of the menopause sequelae is aimed at controlling all the symptoms. This raises the possibility that demedicalization of the menopause might actually improve a woman's experience of this event.

Phytoestrogens

Phytoestrogens are naturally occurring compounds found in plants. They are structurally and functionally similar to 17β oestradiol, the predominant naturally occurring premenopausal oestrogen. They were first identified in the 1930s and their potential biological activity was realized when a species of clover containing phytoestrogens caused infertility in female sheep. Phytoestrogens are found in many different plants, but mainly in legumes, cereals, seed oils and grasses. They produce a very weak oestrogenic effect, competing with the body's oestrogen for the oestrogen receptors. Although there are many different phytoestrogens, the most significant ones in the control of menopausal symptoms are likely to be isoflavones and lignans. Isoflavones are found predominantly in soya beans and soya products whereas lignans are found in oilseeds and cereals.

Diet has long been thought to be the cause of many so-called 'Western diseases', including cancer of the breast, bowel and endometrium as well as cardiovascular disease. This is also true for the menopausal symptoms, as already mentioned, and menopause-related problems. Populations with a high dietary intake of phytoe-strogens have been noted to be associated with a decreased incidence of these diseases and a low incidence of menopausal symptoms. In countries such as Japan, that have diets with high levels of phytoe-strogens, the incidence of these malignancies and menopausal symptoms is significantly lower than in Western countries, suggesting that phytoestrogens may offer a degree of protection. Japanese immigrants to Hawaii adopting a Western lifestyle acquired Western rates of disease within one generation (Smith 1956).

Phytoestrogens behave as both oestrogen agonists and antagonists at oestrogen-receptor level. This explains why the rates of breast, colon and endometrial cancer are lower in areas of high phytoestrogen intake, whereas one might expect the incidence of these diseases to be higher. In postmenopausal women, use of oestrogens without an opposing progestogen increases the risk of endometrial cancer. Prolonged oestrogen exposure is linked to a higher risk of breast cancer, yet breast cancer is less common in populations with a high phytoestrogen intake. The clinical potential for a naturally occurring compound that is selective in its effects is an obvious and also very attractive alternative for menopausal women wanting to avoid pharmacological treatments.

Australia is leading the world in phytoestrogen research. The research done so far into the effects and safety of phytoestrogens looks promising, but extensive clinical trials are still required to confirm their safety and reveal any unwanted side effects, and will perhaps highlight other potential beneficial effects. Even less research has been carried out in women who have had a premature menopause. However, one factor is clear from the epidemiological research to date – that phytoestrogens need to be incorporated into a balanced diet at an early age to confer a protective effect over a lifetime (see Knight & Eden 1995).

Burgen, a bread made from soya flour and linseeds is now available in major supermarkets and has high levels of phytoestrogens. The manufacturers claim that four slices of the bread daily is sufficient to reduce menopausal flush symptomatology. Other breads and phytoestrogen-containing foods or food supplements have become available over the counter and the number of these will probably increase. The daily dose thought to improve menopause symptomatology is 40 mg isoflavones. It is important when buying any alternative remedy or food supplement over the counter to purchase well-known brands where the manufacture and quality of the product are more likely to be better controlled. Unfortunately, women on lower incomes will be disadvantaged by these new products, since phytoestrogen bread is about three times as expensive as an ordinary economy loaf. Phytoestrogen cookery books are also likely to become available.

Complementary therapies

The use of complementary therapies is not new in healthcare; many of the therapies go back hundreds of years. Indeed, massage is instinctive, e.g. rubbing a child's bump better. The use of complementary therapies has increased enormously over the past decade and this is not limited to the UK; it is true too in Europe and the USA. Although there is renewed interest, complementary medicine has always been used in different cultures and countries throughout history. It is hard to explain why so many people should now be turning to complementary therapies, but this may possibly be due to the recognition that orthodox medicine has its limitations and there are many facets of chronic and catastrophic disease that it fails to treat. Indeed, complementary medicine has been described as 'big business' and what was thought to be quackery has become part of accepted practice. More and more people are using complementary therapies, continue to use them and are prepared to pay for them out of their own pocket. More institutions are training new practitioners in complementary medicine and the number of articles on complementary medicine in mainstream medical journals has increased sixfold in the past 30 years.

According to one survey, three out of 10 people have tried complementary medicine. Those who have tried complementary approaches seem to be pleased with the outcome of their treatment. One chiropractor reported that 70% of clients were very satisfied and 60% of clients that went to an osteopath or acupuncturist were pleased with their treatment (Woodham 1994).

A great many different types of complementary therapies exist. There are an increasing number of institutions training would-be practitioners, but so far very few are controlled by legislation. There is little research available to support many of the claims that are made about the different therapies, but gradually more research is being carried out. Most practitioners are self-employed, without the resources or numbers of clients to fund and run trials.

My interest in the use of complementary medicine for the control of menopause problems came from being involved in a menopause support group for four years. Many of the menopausal women who attended the group had used complementary medicines, for a variety of reasons. Over the years, women invited some of their therapists along to the support group meetings so that other members could experience these different therapies. There are a great many different therapies that women might find helpful for the control of their menopausal symptoms. However, there is no evidence that any of the therapies will reduce the long-term risks to the cardiovascular system and bones, except by helping women to make lifestyle changes and therefore reduce some of the other possible risk factors, such as by reducing obesity, introducing healthy eating and stopping smoking.

With vast array of complementary therapies to choose from, it can be difficult to choose an appropriate therapy and therapist. The British Medical Association (BMA) in their 1993 publication suggested that there about 180 different complementary therapies practised in the UK. Despite this, any person considering a complementary approach should read and learn about different therapies to help them choose a therapy that feels right for them. It may not be appropriate to try a particular therapy because of personal recommendation. Some therapies, for instance, necessitate touch and close physical contact with the therapist and some clients would not feel at ease with this. As in orthodox medicine, it is sometimes necessary to try more than one treatment for a particular health problem if the results of the first therapy are disappointing.

Choosing a therapist is also very important. Standards vary enormously, as does training, which may vary from a few weekend courses to a four- or five-year full-time degree. Only osteopaths and chiropractors have a training that is controlled by government legislation, although most of the well-recognized therapies have a governing body that sets training, clinical practice and professional standards. The Royal College of Nursing produced a helpful consumer checklist in 1993, with suggestions from the BMA to help people feel more confident about choosing a therapist. The list identifies many points but includes:

- What are the practitioners' qualifications and how long was the training?
- Is the therapist a member of a recognized, registered body with codes of practice?
- Is the therapy available on the NHS?
- Can the GP delegate your care to the therapist?
- Does the therapist keep the GP informed of any treatment used?
- Is this the most suitable treatment for the condition?
- What is the cost of treatment and how many treatments will be needed?
- Can the patient claim through private health insurance?
- Is the practitioner covered by professional indemnity insurance?

Practitioners who make excessive claims about the success of their treatment or those who suggest that conventional medicine should be discontinued without consulting the GP first, should be avoided. Building up a relationship and a rapport with a practitioner is an important factor in healing, so if the practitioner makes a client feel uncomfortable, another practitioner should be found.

Although there are so many different therapies, they do have certain principles in common. First, they aim to treat the person as a whole, which includes the body, mind and spirit. Second, they believe that the body has its own healing mechanisms, which can be mobilized to restore balance and health to the whole system. Last, people need to be taken in the context of their circumstances and environment and the contributution these can have to ill health.

Most women will find therapies with which they feel comfortable and helpful. In the menopause support group, the therapies that were most commonly used were massage, aromatherapy, reflexology, homeopathy, herbalism (with caution) and acupuncture. However, this list is by no means exhaustive.

Massage

Massage consists of kneading and stroking the body to relieve pain, aid circulation and relax tense muscles. Its main uses are for stress-related conditions, such as insomnia and headaches, together with depression and anxiety, all of which can occur during the menopause and contribute to hot flushes and night sweats. Hippocrates wrote of massage in the fifth century BC and it was also used in ancient Chinese, Egyptian, Roman and Greek cultures. In the West, massage has fallen in and out of favour over the centuries, largely due to the attitude of the church towards indulging the body. However, serious massage has made a comeback in healthcare, largely through the nursing profession, which has always recognized the healing properties of touch.

Massage as we know it today, was developed by a Swedish gymnast, Per Henrik Ling, in the early part of the nineteenth century. There are a variety of massage movements, which include: effleurage – a light, gentle yet firm stroking; petrissage – a firm kneading and rolling of the tissues; and tapotement – hacking, tapping and clapping over the muscles and fleshy parts of the body.

The skin is the body's largest sensory organ – the dermis contains thousands of receptor cells, which react to external stimuli such as heat, cold and pressure, and these messages are then sent to the brain. Gentle stroking can release endorphins, which are the body's own natural painkillers. More vigorous massage can help stretch stiff muscles and joints. Massage can stimulate the circulation, which in turn improves the supply of oxygen and nutrients to the tissues and assist the lymphatics to clear away toxins.

Massage is not a cure for any particular complaint but the feeling of wellbeing created by massage is able to lower the levels of stress hormones. Various trials have examined the effectiveness of massage in the reduction of anxiety, stress, muscular tension and pain relief, although no work has been carried out in menopausal women. Massage can be used in conjunction with other complementary therapies such as aromatherapy, reflexology and shaitsu. Massage is not recommended for people who suffer from phlebitis, thrombosis, varicose veins, tumours, acute back pain or during a fever.

Aromatherapy

This involves the use of essential oils extracted from plants by distillation, for therapeutic effect. The oils are extracted from the leaves, stalks, flowers or roots of plants and are believed to have medicinal properties. The oils are complex chemical compounds and their molecules are thought to enter the bloodstream either through the lungs by inhalation or through the skin. They should not be swallowed. Essential oils can be administered during massage, in a bath or inhaled by adding a few drops to very hot water. How the essential oils work is not entirely understood. The psychological effects of smell are relatively well documented, but how smell can affect the mood, the nervous system and eventually health is still something of a mystery. The oils, which should be of the highest quality, are always diluted before use in a vegetable-based oil such as almond oil. They should always be used with caution as they are potentially toxic compounds. Anyone who is known to be sensitive or to have allergies should always have a patch test first.

The medicinal properties of plants have been recognized for thousands of years. In the Middle ages and Elizabethan period, aromatic oils were popular as medicines and perfumes. It was in the 1920s that the French chemist Rene-Maurice Gattefosse accidentally burnt his hand while working in a perfume factory and applied lavender oil to soothe it. The burn healed well and quickly. Intrigued, he made a study of the therapeutic qualities of plant oils.

Aromatherapy massage is likely to induce states of relaxation, which can reduce anxiety and hot flushes (Hunter & Liao 1996). In addition, some women have informally reported that aromatherapy was helpful in the control of menstrual irregularities, thrush and menopause-related psychological symptoms.

Reflexology

This treatment involves applying pressure to one part of the body, usually the hands or the feet, to promote healing in another part together with a feeling of wellbeing and relaxation. According to reflexologists, every part of our body is reflected in an area of our feet and hands, so that by applying pressure and massaging the soles and toes, energy is unblocked and our natural healing powers enhanced to restore the balance of good health. Although foot massage was used in Egyptian times, reflexology as we know it today was not introduced in the UK until the 1960s. It is easy to learn and simple to perform.

Reflexologists believe that the body is divided into 10 zones that run up from the feet to the head. Within these zones the organs are connected by the flow of energy, and any accessible part of a zone, for example the feet, can be used to treat another part of that zone. This therapy can be organ-specific but can affect the relationship between different organs. If there is an imbalance or blockage of one of these zones, the area of the foot representing this zone becomes tender to touch.

There has been little research on reflexology and early menopause. However, one study looking at its use for premenstrual syndrome showed a 39% improvement in the active group compared to 13.8% in the placebo group (Oleson & Flocco 1993). A study is currently being carried out at the Department of Complementary Medicine, Exeter University, comparing reflexology with general foot massage for women experiencing menopausal symptoms. The preliminary results are promising.

After treatment, reflexologists claim the body has to eliminate many toxins and a healing crisis may occur, resulting in flu-like symptoms, light-headedness, lethargy or altered sleep. The therapeutic potential of reflexology in the menopause may include control of anxiety and stress-related problems, menstrual problems and pain.

Homeopathy

Homeopathy is based on the idea that 'like cures like'. Although this principle was described by Hippocrates in the fifth century BC, it was rediscovered by a German doctor, Samuel Hahnemann, about 200 years ago. The theory on which homeopathy is based is that a substance that causes symptoms of illness in a healthy person can be used to treat similar symptoms in someone who is ill. The purpose of this is to jolt our own self-healing powers, the so-called 'vital force', into action.

Homeopathic remedies are extremely safe. They are derived from animal, vegetable or mineral sources, but are diluted many, many times over so that it is sometimes questionable whether any molecules of the original substance remain. Between each dilution the mixture is shaken vigorously (known as sucussion) so that the cure leaves its 'footprint' in the solution. The weaker the solution the more effective the cure.

Some homeopathic remedies are universal, such as arnica for bruising. However, homeopaths treat each client as an individual, looking at their symptoms, habits and personality traits, so that different remedies are given for the same symptoms in different individuals. Homeopathy must be given time to work and effective treatment may also involve changes in diet and lifestyle with more relaxation and exercise.

Homeopathy is the most widely accepted of all complementary therapies and is available on the NHS, which indeed encompasses several homeopathic hospitals. It is reported to be effective in treating troublesome menopausal symptoms and menstrual problems (Webb 1997), although no research has been done looking at women with an early menopause. It also may be helpful in reducing nausea and improving general health in patients undergoing radiotherapy and chemotherapy, and also for reducing skin tenderness following radiotherapy.

Acupuncture

This is part of traditional Chinese medicine that aims to diagnose illness and promote health by stimulating the body's self-healing powers. Other parts of traditional Chinese medicine include the use of herbs, diet, massage and exercise. The origins of acupuncture have been lost in the mists of time. Acupuncturists believe that the body is permeated by a life force called 'Qi' (pronounce chi), which flows in 12 channels or meridians around the body. Dotted along the meridians are acupuncture points where Qi enters and leaves the body. Acupuncturists believe that an even flow of Qi is essential to health. Traditional Chinese medicine also suggests that there are two opposing forces within the body, Yin and Yang, and a disturbance of flow of Qi leads to a disturbance of Yin and Yang, resulting in ill health, both physical and emotional. Acupuncture involves the insertion of fine, sterile needles into these acupuncture points, of which there are about 365, to free the flow of Qi and thus bring the body back into harmony.

Acupuncture has become increasingly accepted by the medical profession over the past few decades, although the existence of Qi and meridians cannot be explained within the parameters of Western medicine. Over 700 trials have been undertaken on the effects of acupuncture on the menopause, but only one in English. This study showed that acupuncture improved flush symptomatology, and the improvement continued for three months after the final treatment (Wyon et al. 1995). Acupuncture has been found to be helpful in some people for making lifestyle changes, such as reducing smoking or controlling obesity, which are both important in reducing the risk of heart disease. There is limited availability under the NHS; a number of GPs are trained in acupuncture.

Alcohol, hot baths, strenuous exercise (including sex) and large meals are to be avoided before and after treatment.

Herbalism

Herbalism is the use of medicinal plants to treat disease and promote good health. It is the precursor to our modern pharmacopoeia; examples include digoxin from foxgloves and salicylic acid (similar to aspirin) from meadow sweet. About a quarter of all pharmaceutical preparations contain an active plant ingredient. However, herbalists rarely isolate the active ingredient from the plant and use the whole plant, believing that the remedy works through a delicate balance of all the constituents in the plant. These work together to enhance its action, make it safe and minimize side effects. In the UK, the role of the herbalist was recognized in the 1968 Medicines Act, which makes provision for potentially potent herbal medicines to be prescribed by a professional herbalist. In 1985, the World Health Organisation recognized the importance of herbalism in meeting health needs. The BMA describes herbalism as a 'discrete clinical entity'. In some European countries it is integrated into the health-care system.

Herbalism was used in the ancient civilizations of Egypt, China, Persia and India. Hippocrates and Galen practised herbalism and their learning filtered back through Europe with the crusaders. In England, Culpeper wrote a book on herbal treatments in 1649.

Clinical research supports claims made for many herbs, such as the use of garlic to lower cholesterol and the effect of St John's Wort to treat depression. Herbalism can be used for most illnesses, although patients with illnesses requiring surgery or diagnostic tests should be referred immediately to medical doctor and those with musculoskeletal conditions to a chiropractor or osteopath. Herbalism can be effective in chronic conditions such as migraine, arthritis and skin complaints. Other conditions include premenstrual and menopausal problems, depression, and problems of the respiratory, digestive and circulatory systems. The remedies used may be tinctures applied to the skin (made by steeping the herb in alcohol) or they may be ingested as tablets, defusions and concoctions. Creams, lotions and ointments are all taken externally. The quality of the herbs used in different preparations, together with source, purity and dosage, can vary and consumers should stick to well-known brands.

Contrary to popular belief, not all herbs are without side effects and it is essential to consult a qualified herbalist. Indeed, some herbs may be strongly contraindicated. For example, in women with a history of breast cancer; any herb with oestrogen-like properties may potentially have a deleterious effect.

In 1978, Germany established Commission E to review the safety and efficacy of over 1400 herbal drugs but only about 300 had their effects supported by clinical trials and approved. However, many herbs are available for improvement of menopausal symptoms, the list below is not conclusive but includes some of the commonly reported herbs.

- Black Cohosh is thought to have an oestrogen-like action; it is thought by some to be a rich source of phytoestrogens. Three randomised studies suggest that Black Cohosh is effective in the treatment of flushes and the psychological symptoms of menopause. Commission E recommended that it should not be taken for more than six months, but in the studies the safety data were good, with a frequency of adverse events similar to those of a placebo (Taylor 1997; Ernst 1999).
- Dong Quai is often given to treat hot flushes and almost any female gynaecological complaint. Dong Quai contains a number of derivatives and also an essential oil. There is some concern that the oil contains a carcinogenic compound, therefore more research is needed on this product (Israel & Youngkin 1997).
- Chaste Tree is a herb widely suggested for menopausal symptoms including hot flushes. It is considered to be the best herb for the control of menopausal mood swings and is popular in Europe for treating premenstrual syndrome (PMS) and menopause (Israel & Youngkin 1997). Research has found it to be effective in treating PMS but its effect on the menopause at any age is not established.
- Ginseng is considered by many to be the wonder herb, used by the Chinese for over 5000 years. It is believed to increase oestrogen levels and has been reported to produce mastalgia in post-menopausal women. The herb is thought to be generally safe, except in women who are advised against taking oestrogen (Hendrix 1997). However, there is no published evidence of its efficacy for perimenopausal and menopausal problems. Ginseng is to undergo safety checks with the US National Toxicology Programme shortly.
- Sage is said to relieve hot flushes and decrease perspiration (Israel & Youngkin 1997). It is safe in small amounts in cooking but

larger amounts used over a period of time may induce psychological and physical side effects.

- St John's Wort has been shown in a number of clinical trials to significantly improve mild to moderate depression compared with a placebo (Harrar & Sommer 1994). It was relatively free from side effects, the most common being dizziness, gastrointestinal symptoms, confusion and tiredness. The recommended duration of therapy is unknown.

- Feverfew has been shown in a number of randomised placebo-controlled trials to have a beneficial effect on migraines, although the studies were not specifically undertaken in menopausal women. Side effects are few and reversible; they include mouth ulcers and gastrointestinal symptoms with extended use (Ernst 1999).

- Kava has been shown to be effective in the control of anxiety in seven randomised placebo-controlled, double-blind trials. The safety profile was good and there were only mild side effects, which included gastrointestinal symptoms, restlessness, drowsiness, tremor, headache and tiredness (Ernst 1999). However, this herb is to undergo safety checks by the US National Toxicology Programme.

- Valerian is widely marketed over the counter as a remedy for insomnia. A number of studies have been undertaken, of which half have shown it to be effective in improving sleep.

Natural progesterone cream

A number of natural progesterone creams are available via mail order or from health shops. The creams are mainly derived from wild yams, which are well known to contain progesterone-like compounds. There are claims that it is progesterone that is the forgotten hormone in menopause treatment and it has been claimed that progesterone cream can treat menopausal symptoms and reverse the effects of osteoporosis (Lee 1990). These claims have not been confirmed by other researchers. Many women who use progesterone cream have felt extremely well on it. However, little research has been conducted on progesterone cream and more is still required to clarify its effects. At the moment it is an unlicensed product that is sold as a dietary supplement.

A trial comparing one progesterone cream, Progest, to a placebo and oral progesterone tablets found that there was very little difference in the body's progesterone levels between the placebo and the active Progest cream (Cooper et al. 1998). Until there are more data available it is difficult to support its use. There is concern over the safety of its use in women who have been omitting the progestogen part of their HRT and replacing it with a progesterone cream. The levels of progesterone absorbed are unlikely to be effective in protecting the endometrium and if this continued over time it could lead to an increased risk endometrial cancer.

Simple self-help measures

There is evidence that a high calcium intake during childhood and adolescence, with regular exercise, improves peak adult bone mass (Bronner 1994). Bone mass peaks in both sexes in the mid-thirties and then begins a slow ageing-related bone loss. However, in women there is an additional and accelerated period of bone loss after the menopause. In some women who have a premature menopause before their thirties and before adult bone mass peaks, bone loss may begin to occur at a time when it should still be being laid down. The risk of osteoporosis is dependent on the amount of bone mass laid down and the rate at which it is lost. Calcium intake does seem to have a beneficial effect on bone turnover (Dawson-Hughes et al. 1990). However, as women get older they absorb calcium less efficiently from the gut, so proportionally more needs to be consumed. For adult women the daily recommended intake is 1000 mg, but this rises to 1500 mg daily in women over 45 years and menopausal women not on HRT (see Table 10.1 for calcium contents of food). The best source of calcium is from dairy products, but the consumption of milk products has dropped over the past decade. Many women think of dairy products as fattening. However, skimmed milk contains marginally more calcium than full-cream products and contains fewer calories than an ordinary cola drink. Some milks are fortified with additional calcium, which is helpful for women struggling to meet the daily allowance, but some women may still need to take a calcium supplement. Many such supplements are available, and some GPs may prescribe them. If buying them over the counter, a well-known brand should be chosen and the amount of calcium contained in each tablet noted. Some tablets have a low calcium content and several tablets need to be taken daily (Table 10.1).

A good calcium intake will not necessarily prevent osteoporosis, but it does help reduce the rate of bone loss, particularly in women

Table 10.1: The calcium content of foods

Food	Serving	Calcium content (mg)
Cheddar cheese	100 mg	720
Sesame seeds	100 mg	670
Canned sardines (with bones)	100 mg	550
Dried figs	100 mg	250
Almonds	100 mg	240
Yoghurt	100 mg	190
Watercress	100 mg	170
Skimmed milk	100 ml	124
Semi-skimmed milk	100 ml	122
Ice cream, non-diary vanilla	100 mg	120
Whole milk	100 ml	119
White bread	100 mg	110
Canned salmon	100 mg	93
Fromage frais, plain	100 mg	89
Plain cottage cheese	100 mg	73
Peanuts	100 mg	60
Wholemeal bread	100 mg	54
Baked beans	100 mg	53
Spring cabbage	100 mg	42
Broccoli	100 mg	40

who previously had a poor calcium intake. Studies in turn have shown that an increased calcium intake in older women can reduce fracture risk. Other dietary factors that are important include an adequate protein and caloric intake, as malnutrition and low body mass index are both associated with a reduced bone mass. Smoking, alcohol and caffeine all have a detrimental effect on calcium absorption and metabolism and should be discouraged or their intake moderated (Clunie 1994). Excessive alcohol intake is associated with osteoporosis, partially due to a toxic effect of the alcohol on osteoblasts, the cells in the bone that replace and build up bone mass. Excessive alcohol is also associated with malnutrition. There is a link between smoking and osteoporosis and therefore giving up smoking is something that women with premature menopause can do to help themselves.

Vitamin D helps calcium absorption from the gut. In the UK, most people gain sufficient vitamin D from exposure to sunlight, although it is also available from foods such as fortified margarines, cereals, milk, egg yolks and salt-water fish. However, some Asian women, and institutionalized women, do develop vitamin D deficiency (due to the lack of exposure to sunlight) and supplementation has been shown to reduce fracture risk (Chapuy et al. 1992).

Multivitamin and mineral supplements

Multivitamin and mineral supplements are widely available in health food shops and chemists, and some are specifically targeted for the menopausal woman. Vitamins and minerals are naturally occurring substances required in very small amounts for the normal functioning of the body and are essential for life. There are approximately 13 vitamins and 25 minerals essential in an average diet. The vitamins can be broadly divided into two groups: the fat-soluble minerals (vitamins A, D and E), which dissolve in fat and can be stored in our bodies; and the water-soluble vitamins (vitamins B and C), which dissolve in water and cannot be stored. Because vitamins B and C cannot be stored, a regular intake is required.

Minerals are inorganic, non-living substances that are derived from the soil in which plants grow. They are also divided into two categories: those of which we only need a minute amount, called trace elements, such as selenium; and those which are needed in larger quantities, referred to as minerals, such as iron and calcium.

The rationale behind these supplements is to provide the vitamins and minerals that may be helpful in meeting the special needs of women with early menopause or that may be deficient in the diet because of lack of bioavailability, poor absorption or due to dietary deficiencies. For instance, vitamin B is involved in the release of energy from food, thus a boost of vitamin B complex is aimed at improving energy levels, as tiredness can be a particular problem at the menopause. Some recent research has indicated that vitamin E supplementation has a cardioprotective effect, which may be beneficial as the risk of heart disease increases after the menopause. Folic acid and vitamin B[6] have been shown to have an advantageous effect on the homocysteine levels, which are an additional risk factor for coronary heart disease. Lifestyle factors can affect requirements for minerals and vitamins. Caffeine, alcohol and smoking decrease the absorption of these nutrients and thus increase the requirements. Although supplementation may provide short-term reassurance, women should consider reducing their intake of these stimulants.

The need for certain vitamins is also linked to our metabolic rate, which can be speeded up by vigorous exercise or stress. This creates an increased demand for the vitamin B group vitamins involved in energy production.

Some early studies showed that vitamin supplementation improved flush symptomatology (McLaren 1949), although more recent studies did not support these findings. Anecdotally, some women have reported an improvement in vasomotor symptoms with a multivitamin and mineral preparation. The daily levels for improvement are unknown and may depend on the quality of individual diets. This area warrants further research.

Oil of evening primrose

Many women take oil of evening primrose (OEP) for a variety of complaints. The oil contains an essential fatty acid called gammalinolenic acid (GLA). This is converted to prostaglandins, which are hormone-like substances involved in many normal body functions. Many studies have been carried out on OEP and have shown it to be effective in the control of breast tenderness and helpful in premenstrual syndrome. However, a well-controlled study has been published on the effect of OEP on menopausal symptoms, which showed that it did not improve menopausal hot flushes (Chenoy et al. 1994).

Simple measures to improve menopausal symptoms

There are a number of simple measures that some women find helpful when coping with the troublesome symptoms, particularly hot flushes and night sweats. These include avoiding anything that acts as a trigger for the flushes and then action to make them less problematic when they occur.

Well-known triggers for flushes include alcohol, caffeine, spicy food, tobacco and stressful situations. Women who experience flushes often find it helpful to wear several layers of thin clothing. Layers can easily be removed when the flush occurs and then replaced after the flush episode, when many women feel cold. A well-ventilated room during both day and night often increases comfort. Night sweats can be miserable if profuse perspiration means that sheets have to be changed during the night. Some women find sleeping on a towel or wearing a lightweight towelling dressing gown can avoid changing bedclothes at night. Choice of bedclothes can also become problematic as women become incompatible with their partners through feeling hot at night. Some women have found it easier to use single duvets, which is common on the continent, and to have a cooler one than their partner. Counselling and stress management can also be helpful when stress is a trigger for flushes and relaxation with cognitive-behavioural treatment has been found to be effective (Hunter & Liao 1996).

Exercise

Regular exercise is important for a number of reasons: it protects against heart disease and conserves bone mass, as well as providing a feeling of wellbeing and reducing some menopausal symptoms.

There is some evidence to suggest that women who exercise regularly are less troubled by menopausal hot flushes and experience less depression and insomnia around the menopause (Payer 1991). There are no guidelines to suggest exactly how much exercise is needed, but any exercise should to be tailored to a woman's fitness and carried out on several occasions each week.

Exercise is vital for the health of the skeleton. Regular weight-bearing and muscle-strengthening exercise such as walking is important for bone density (Prince et al. 1991). Total immobilization, even for short periods, results in bone loss. It has been shown that over an 18-month period there is a significant increase in bone mineral density in those undertaking weight-bearing exercise three times weekly (Heinonen et al. 1996). However, young women who exercise excessively so that periods stop are increasing their risk of osteoporosis because oestrogen levels become lowered and bone loss occurs at a time in a young woman's life when bone mass should still be increasing. In a young woman who has a premature menopause before her mid-thirties – before peak adult bone mass has been reached – it is important that she takes exercise and has a sufficient calcium intake. These are needed to maximize the amount of bone that is laid down, which in turn reduces the risk of the bone mass dropping to osteoporotic levels in later life. The aim is to prevent osteoporosis, to maximize bone mass and to reduce bone loss, since once bone mass has been lost it can not be replaced.

Lifestyle changes for the prevention of coronary heart disease

There are many factors that affect the risk of coronary heart disease (CHD). Some of these factors cannot be changed, such as age, sex, premature menopause and family history of CHD. There is evidence that modification of other lifestyle-related risk factors are effective in reducing the risk of CHD. These changes are beneficial for reducing the overall risk and also in patients with established disease (Pyorala et al. 1994).

There are three main areas that are well-recognized as risk factors for CHD: smoking, high blood pressure and high cholesterol. In the so-called 'Western culture', a diet rich in saturated fats and calories, tobacco smoking and physical inactivity have increased the rate of CHD in these populations. These lifestyles cause changes within the body that lead to CHD, such as the formation of atheroma in blood vessels and the increased tendency for thrombosis. There is also a genetic influence on the blood lipids and blood pressure but lifestyle changes do continue to make a contribution to the progress of the disease. Favourable changes in lifestyle reduce the risk of CHD.

Any person making these changes needs to understand the responsibility he or she has in making them so they are effective in the long term. Although healthcare professionals can help highlight areas that need modification, it is up to each individual to implement them effectively.

A varied diet that provides all the necessary vitamins and minerals is required to maintain a healthy body. Other recommendations include a low total fat intake, high fibre, low sugar and low salt. Dietary salt can increase high blood pressure. A low-fat diet can reduce the more harmful low-density lipoproteins (LDLs) in the blood. In addition, fibre and complex carbohydrates from vegetable sources may have a protective role. Obesity has an adverse effect on several risk factors for CHD as it is a nutrition-related disorder.

Smoking is responsible for 50% of all avoidable deaths, of which half are due to cardiovascular disease. The adverse effect is related to the amount of tobacco smoked and the duration of smoking. Even though smoking is harmful in both sexes, the effect may be stronger in women. Smoking has a greater impact on the risk of CHD in populations with high LDL levels. It enhances the rate of atheroma formation and in some people it can take up to 10 years after stopping smoking for the risk level to return to a non-smoker's level.

Alcohol

Alcohol tends to increase the levels of high-(HDLs) lipoproteins in the blood, which can be protective against coronary heart disease. This beneficial effect is present in moderate drinkers (1–3 units of alcohol daily) and non-drinkers have a higher risk than moderate drinkers. However, heavy drinkers increase their risk of high blood pressure, strokes and sudden death. Other adverse health effects tend to offset the beneficial effects of alcohol.

Physical inactivity

There is strong evidence that a sedentary lifestyle increases CHD risk. Regular physical activity reduces LDL levels, overweight and reduces blood pressure. Maintenance of regular physical activity is important for cardiovascular health and is protective against strenuous exercise acting as a trigger for a cardiovascular incident.

Blood pressure

Blood pressure has been shown to increase CHD, cardiac failure and strokes. Lifestyle changes that reduce blood pressure include reducing dietary salt intake, relaxation, reduction in weight and alcohol use, and increasing physical activity.

Conclusion

Women who have a premature menopause need to be especially aware of the health risks of long-term menopausal consequences and what they can do to help themselves. Although there is concern for immediate relief from menopausal symptoms and much can be done using lifestyle changes, every effort needs to be made to ensure good long-term health without the use of conventional medicine. With personal involvement and long-term commitment, many women find it helpful to control aspects of their health and wellbeing using complementary treatments and lifestyle changes. These treatments warrant more research, and the most appropriate treatment for each problem in each woman should be focused upon.

Chapter 11
Self-help and support groups

LIH-MEI LIAO, ZELDA ABRAMSON AND
CATHERINE CORP

Many women with premature menopause express a sense of alienation and isolation. Feelings of being cut off from others can further weaken self-esteem. Groups can provide a way of sharing and normalizing the experience of premature menopause. The importance of theme-centred support groups has long been recognized, but they are not for everyone. Although one can never completely comprehend the feelings of another person, those who have been through a similar predicament can empathise with each other. The more similar the concerns, the more likely the group members are to feel that their particular worries are addressed. Groups operate as a support system, enabling recognition of others in the same situation. Through involvement in the tasks of group building and sustaining the group system, members become freer over time to disclose their pain and to carry over the gains made within the group into their social world. In this way self-esteem can be restored, expectations of self and others modified, and the need for withdrawal mitigated.

Groups can provide less threatening settings in which to ask the questions that members may feel inhibited about asking a physician. This may help to improve communication with doctors at a later date. Sharing knowledge increases control and participation in decision making, particularly in relation to treatments such as hormone replacement therapy (HRT) and/or egg donation, while simultaneously counteracting tendencies towards self-recrimination. Humour can be used to lighten the tragic quality of feelings of loss and emphasize ingenuity in the face of what can be perceived as unwarranted prying by insensitive outsiders. For longer-term issues, decisions to seek out further psychological help may become more positively framed.

Support groups can serve an educational and empowerment function as well as being a forum for information exchange. Women can learn that they are not insane or abnormal and that they can help themselves and each other. They can facilitate coping strategies, helping women come to terms with often painful and conflicting feelings.

In this chapter, three different types of group are highlighted. The first emphasizes positive coping strategies that can emerge from even time-limited groups, where confidentiality is strictly maintained and there is sensitive management of the conflicting needs and demands of group members. The second outlines the emotional and informational support ongoing groups can offer. The third stretches the definition of group to include a worldwide support group that can be found over the Internet.

An eight-session group psychological intervention

LIH-MEI LIAO

The aim of this section is to describe the process, content and outcome of a brief psychological intervention for a group of four women who have experienced premature menopause. The group took place within the setting of the outpatient menopause clinic in an inner London NHS teaching hospital, serving a socially mixed catchment area. A clinical psychology service offering assessment and treatment for menopausal women is carried out in parallel to a medical clinic. The service offers mainly short-term, focused work. Women with psychological concerns relating to menopause can either refer themselves or are referred by their physician.

The need for developing such a group was identified from separate processes. A recent questionnaire study carried out by a trainee and the author had identified considerable psychological difficulty in relation to premature menopause; the development of cost-effective means for alleviating distress was clearly indicated. The work with individual women in the past had highlighted the issue of social isolation; it was therefore felt that brief group interventions might partly answer some of these needs. By chance, five women with premature menopause were referred to me within a short period, although one did not take up her appointment. Of the four who followed through their referral, two of the woman were self-referrals and the other two were referred by their medical consultant.

Objectives of the group intervention

* to provide a context in which women who have experienced premature menopause can feel safe to discuss their experience and its impact upon their lives
* to offer information about the condition
* to enable the participants to reappraise how they view themselves and their future, thereby to further the process of adaptation and adjustment.

The participants

Three of the four women had been diagnosed recently, while the fourth had known about her premature menopause for over four years. The names and identifiable details of the women have been changed.

Clare is 33 years old, single and white British. She is happy in her work as an administrator and lives alone in her own home. Her periods started at the age of 14 and were irregular from the beginning, with occasional long intervals of up to a year between periods. Medical investigations in her mid-twenties did not provide evidence for early menopause. Her last spontaneous menstrual period was at age 27. Subsequently she took the oral contraceptive pill for a year. At the age of 32, Clare had surgery for an ovarian cyst. During surgery, her ovaries were noted to be small and premature ovarian failure (POF) was suspected. This was immediately confirmed by the raised gonadotrophin and low serum oestrogen measurements.

Yasmine is 37 and single. She identified her family background as British Asian. She and her siblings were born and brought up in

Edinburgh, where the rest of the family still live and where she said she still has a strong supportive network. Yasmine's mother and two sisters have all experienced premature menopause.

At the time she referred herself to the service Yasmine was in the middle of a number of life transitions. Her relationship of three year's standing had broken up. While in the relationship, she had become pregnant and had terminated the pregnancy due to uncertainty surrounding the partnership. Upon its ending, Yasmine moved out to a friend's house as a temporary measure. She started to experience symptoms, which she attributed to stress. Her diagnosis was confirmed soon after. In the meantime, her fixed-term work contract was due to end and she was having to reconsider work positions.

Ayshe is 40 years old, lives on her own and has worked on and off as a freelance private tutor. She identified herself as Iraqi. At the time of the group, she was struggling with her attempt to stop smoking, as it interfered with what to her was the most important activity of her life – her singing.

Ayshe described her background as 'difficult' with both parents having had psychiatric problems. She came to Britain to study when she was 18 years old. At the age of 36, she went home to Iraq to attend her mother's funeral. She experienced severe physical symptoms, which she then associated with the emotional trauma and now knows to be hot flushes. She has had many unsatisfactory relationships with men. She has also had contact with the psychiatric services, mainly on account of addiction problems.

Sheila is 36 years of age. She has been with the same partner for nine years but described their relationship as 'uncertain' following the diagnosis of premature menopause. She felt as if she was coping with two losses. Furthermore, although she was not unhappy with work as a teacher, she did not see herself 'throwing life into work'. She said that she had suddenly felt the need to 'review' her entire life. She felt that she had lost a lot of confidence following her diagnosis but also attributed this to her weight gain. Upon receiving her diagnosis, she found out that her mother had also experienced early menopause and was aghast that this had never been mentioned. Sheila did not want a baby 'just for the sake of it' but had felt pressured by the threat of losing the opportunity. She asked about the possibility of freezing her own eggs.

The therapists

The therapists were me, a clinical psychologist specializing in problems in relation to reproductive endocrinology, and Victoria Byram, who was in the final stage of her doctoral programme in clinical psychology.

A developing framework for the group

Premature menopause breaks many social rules. Many women feel marginalized as a result of their diagnosis and its consequences. Several aspects of premature menopause require psychological adjustment, including infertility during normative child-bearing years, transition to menopausal status before mid-life, increased risks to future health and consequently the recommended long-term use of HRT. For younger women, these aspects of their life place them in a socially deviant position and can pose a serious threat to their self-identity. Sociocultural as well as psychological frameworks are useful for making sense of these issues and to achieve other aims: to increase knowledge about the condition and healthcare, and to mobilize personal resources in order to maximize self-help and psychosocial adaptation.

While this type of therapeutic work can be carried out with individuals, a group approach can have many advantages. Group work has multiple origins and has been developed in different contexts; much has been written about it and it is not the remit of this chapter to debate the issues. Our particular structure combined the components of self-help health groups (Robinson 1980) and principles of behaviour change (Salkovskis 1998).

In the context of our group, sharing is explicitly recognized as a key feature of the process. The rationale behind it is that through sharing, a range of perspectives on the problem or a degree of deconstruction is achieved. This involves initially concentrating on the problem, and it is not unusual for participants to say at this stage that they feel worse. However, the acknowledgement and validation, together with additional information, self-monitoring and goal planning, may eventually enable participants to problem solve, such as in the areas of nutritional improvement, social assertion and so on. These processes also contribute towards another level of deconstruction: destigmatization. The shifting of perceptions achieved with others who share the condition help to disperse perceived social discredibility of the participants and their shared problems. This part of the process is sometimes referred to as 'differential association' (Killilea 1976), which emphasizes the participants' mutual reinforcement of self-concepts or normality and hastens their departure from the previous conception of themselves as deviant.

Themes of group sessions

- Session 1 – Introductions
- Session 2 – Premature menopause: current explanations and your experience
- Session 3 – Medical treatment and self-help
- Session 4 – Fertility issues
- Session 5 – Sexuality and relationships
- Session 6 – Communication
- Session 7 – Planning for the future
- Session 8 – Individual follow-up session

Structure of group sessions

Each of the sessions focused on a particular aspect of premature menopause and followed a format designed to maximize discussion.

- Review of past week and agreed task
- Introducing current sessional theme
- Questions and information giving
- Facilitated discussion
- Summary of discussion
- Handout on points of information
- Agreed task before next session

Planned evaluation of the group

The eighth session was an individual session that took place two months after the final group session and followed a semi-structured interview format. The women were asked to review what had and had not changed for them, what they felt were the ways forward for them, and to make suggestions for future groups. In addition, they were given two standardized measures of global psychological well-being before and after. The Center of Epidemiologic Studies – Depression Scale (CES-DS) (Radloff 1977) was used to assess current depressive symptomatology. In addition, the Satisfaction

with Life Scale (SWLS) (Diener et al. 1985) was used to assess positive wellbeing. These particular scales had been used in a previous
study with women who have experienced premature menopause
(Liao et al. 1999) and would enable comparison.

Summary of group process

As the group was to be short-term, there was implicit pressure to
build up the momentum quickly. The participants soon started to
contribute to the discussions, helped by the presence of a structure
and the small size of the group. As far as enabling a greater level of
disinhibition was concerned, there were safety issues for a short-term
intervention in which the participants were to meet only seven times.

The boundaries of the group were clarified at the beginning. As
therapists, we saw our roles as ensuring that the group took place,
enabling equitable participation as far as possible, and making
meaningful connections of the rich content in each session as guided
by social and psychological frameworks. It was made explicit to the
participants that they had not entered into group psychotherapy. We
also did not give medical advice but offered current available information – conflicting and consensus – where possible, and passed
questions that we could not answer to the relevant expert (e.g.
medical doctor, dietitian).

The usual ground rules were proposed and agreed on in the
introductory session. For example, the women were asked not to
make contact with each other outside the sessions for the duration
of the group, in order to avoid suballiances, which could make
others feel excluded. While each woman was her own expert and
all her views were valid and important in our context, they were
informed that they were not expected to disclose what felt uncomfortable for them at any particular time. Confidentiality issues
were also dealt with at the beginning. As regular attendance was
important not only for the individual but for all the others, the
women were asked to make known any particular difficulty with
this and to propose an alternative time for the sessions and seek
consensus should they wish. At this point, Yasmine tentatively
suggested that the sessions be moved to the evening. This was
readily agreed to.

It was not surprising that the participants were at their most reti-
cent early on. Sheila was the last person to introduce herself in the

first session but the first to acknowledge her anxiety about coming to the group. The subsequent surrounding nods conveyed similar feelings. At the end of the third session, however, Clare mentioned how quickly the sessions came to an end. At this point, Sheila asked to extend the future sessions by another quarter of an hour. This was echoed by others and subsequently taken up.

Each group session ended with the participants agreeing on a personal task related to the sessional theme. This was to be accomplished before the following session in which they would feed back on how they had got on, what the obstacles might have been and whether the rest of the group could make useful suggestions for the individual. An example of this is that at the end of third session each individual agreed on a healthy eating or exercise goal, such as to explore the local gym facilities, eat breakfast or have a piece of fruit every day. Ayshe laughed embarrassingly when the idea was first introduced: 'Oh look at all the homework they have for us!' While each of the actions might not have been significant in itself, it was felt that the practice of systematic and thoughtful planning was important in the process of problem solving.

Summary of discussion content across sessions

The summary is organized into themes and does not follow the sequence of the sessions or the order in which the points were raised.

Circumstances of the diagnosis and reactions to it

The women received their diagnosis under different circumstances. All of them were shocked; none reported positive aspects to the way they received the information.

Ayshe's diagnosis was revealed to her in unusual circumstances. Four years ago at the age of 36, she went home to Iraq for her mother's funeral. At a social gathering, she experienced acute vasomotor symptoms. A 70-year-old woman pointed out that she was in the menopause. Ayshe quickly saw a doctor who confirmed the diagnosis and prescribed herbal treatment for her 'wild hot flushes'. At that point, she was left believing that the condition was reversible. When she returned to Britain, she saw her own doctor and started taking HRT.

Clare's diagnosis was revealed to her shortly after the surgery to remove her cyst. Her reaction was marked by confusion:

I was still feeling woosy from the anaesthetic. The consultant came round and told me that I was menopausal. He gave me HRT and said start taking it right away ... it still doesn't make any sense, no one in my family has had anything like this.

Yasmine was a quieter member of the group but was able to voice similar feelings when Sheila expressed her anger about the way she received her diagnosis:

I got a letter a few days later telling me about egg donation. But I knew I was still fertile.

Yasmine felt particularly traumatized by being told 'in the same breath' that she must be prepared to pay at least £3000 for ovum donation and IVF treatment if she wanted a child, again before she was able to accept that she was infertile. She said:

Afterwards I just walked around in a daze not knowing what to do with myself. This sort of carried on...I knew I wanted children and immediately felt the pressure of finding a partner and going for natural conception right away. I feel I was forced to accomplish this huge psychological leap in no time at all.

Sheila acknowledged her hostile feelings towards her mother (who also had early menopause) for having 'passed it on' and for failing to prepare her for it; while Clare expressed gratitude towards her mother for her support. Several of the women felt that their menopause might have been brought forward by traumatic life events.

Physical health issues

Clinical management tends to focus on the medical aspects of menopause, such as vasomotor and urogenital symptoms, and future risks of osteoporosis and cardiovascular disease. For younger women becoming menopausal, the indication for long-term HRT is deemed clear. None of the women in the group had been asked about their feelings about being medicated for life or given reassurance. They also felt that there was no systematic attempt by health professionals to address their health concerns and the perceived threat to bodily integrity.

Two of the women in this group were on HRT and two were not, although their views were far from polarized. Whatever their decision, all of the women were interested in finding out more about alternative options and self-help.

Ayshe said that she was not happy to have hormones and had experimented with stopping but had now become resigned to it. The reason she gave was:

> I tried to do without them, I came off for three months, did my hot flushes come back, they were unbelievable, I felt so ill.

She had to balance the benefits against her various side effects:

> The first one gave me terrible symptoms, I had the worst PMT ever.

During the time of the group, Ayshe was trying a third HRT regimen, which later proved to be successful in not causing serious side effects.

While she objected to the way her HRT was initially prescribed, Clare had no problem with following medical recommendations and was prepared to take it indefinitely. Her greater acceptance was possibly related to two factors. She had not experienced any side effects, and she was concerned about future health problems. For example she said:

> This [menopause] has been going on silently in my body without my knowing, and I think, what else is going on inside that I don't know about?

Both Sheila and Yasmine have declined taking HRT and have sought homeopathic options, about which all of the women were keen to find out more. They alluded to the view that widespread use of HRT is not only good for women but may have sociopolitical implications. Sheila said:

> How did women used to manage? My grandmother seemed to have had early menopause, she's in her eighties, fit as a fiddle... They all tell you that you must have this, and this is good for you, good for who?

However, both she and Yasmine said that they would reconsider HRT from time to time.

The women asked about the effectiveness of homeopathic options. It had to be pointed out to them that perhaps due to cultural reasons, alternative treatments have remained marginal in Western societies and consequently have not had the same opportunities for scientific evaluation as orthodox medicines. There is, however, anecdotal support for some remedies (see Chapter 10 for a discussion of non-medical approaches). The importance of being in control of their healthcare was emphasized and that if it meant seeking out other remedies, the process itself can be psychologically significant. The women also gave each other strategies for asking questions and for making the most of their future consultations with health professionals.

The evidence for the importance of healthy eating and regular exercise was more scientifically established and these were discussed in some detail. Sheila was keen to pursue exercise to reduce health risks as well as to lose weight. Yasmine did not habitually have dairy products in her diet and other group members were able to contribute useful suggestions on how she could have sufficient calcium in her diet.

Infertility

Motherhood is central to a woman's identity and provides a major context in which women live and through which they relate to others. Childlessness places a woman in an isolated position of social non-conformity. The women grieved the loss of what they had always taken for granted as a primary life goal.

Sheila said in the very first session that she believed she 'could still get pregnant'. She voiced the difficulty of knowing if she would ever have wanted a child should the choice always be there. She asked about the freezing of ovarian tissue and, when informed that the techniques were experimental at the time, she was critical of the limitations of modern medicine:

> They don't know anything; they can't give you any help at all.

On the subject of ovum donation, Clare said:

> It wouldn't be my child, not really. What for? Why not just adopt? Or maybe I will, I don't know. I will never have MY child anyway. I thought I would be, like everyone else, married, have a family. If it's not going to happen, what am I going to do now?

The need for alternative life goals was echoed by Sheila. She said she had always wanted to travel. She was positive about the suggestion that she worked towards allowing herself the equivalent of 'maternity leave' to travel.

Ayshe was the only one who directly challenged the view that 'parenthood is a must for everyone', and added:

> I haven't wanted to be in the menopause but I know I can't look after children. I'm enough problem for me. [laughter] We're brainwashed into wanting children, quite frankly some people shouldn't; I have friends, they all complained, they have no life, they've really changed, they're always feeling guilty, feeling resentful, tired.

She was the only group member who expressly did not wish for a child, regardless of whether or not she was able to. This definitive decision was not shared by the others. However, Yasmine and Sheila both voiced that, while the loss of their fertility was a major aspect of early menopause, the 'bombardment' of untimely information on assisted reproduction gave the message that they should want children. It felt ironic when Clare said that she had previously attended a meeting of a support network for early menopause in which she felt isolated:

> It felt like a springboard for information and discussion about egg donation, and I don't even have a partner, so I just listened.

As most of the women in the current group were not in a position to consider pregnancy, they felt that a forum addressing other existential issues had been lacking.

Menopause and its psychological sequelae

In our culture, menopause is subject to ageist and sexist stereotyping, which can have a self-fulfilling impact (Liao & Hunter 1998). For example, a common belief is that women become unattractive, asexual, and suffer both physically and mentally after menopause. Such negative social stereotypes can contribute to low self-esteem and can be challenged in a group format. Younger women are particularly negative about menopause (Bowles 1986), and such negative beliefs can contribute to symptom severity (Avis & McKinlay 1991) and depressed mood (Hunter 1992). Since health professionals can be even more negative about menopause than their female patients (Cowan et al. 1985; Liao et al. 1994), there may be a risk for emotional distress to be misattributed to menopause, when other factors are also relevant. The group offered the opportunity for discussing various deep-seated fears about menopause and to explore the evidence for and against these negative assumptions.

When these four women first met, they expressed their surprise as to how young their fellow participants looked. Ayshe particularly remarked on Clare's youthful appearance. They were all able to laugh at their expectation of meeting a group of more aged women.

As there is a prevailing belief that hormonal changes in women cause psychological problems, there was some confusion about whether their mood state was related to the physiological menopause, their reaction to being menopausal, or life in general. For instance, Ayshe had had major psychological difficulties while she was still in the premenopause. Yet in one of the sessions she attributed all her current difficulties to the physiological menopause:

> It gets worse and worse, I feel that my body has taken over, one day I feel normal, another day I can hardly get myself out of bed, they tell you take medicine and you're fine, but your body has changed forever, that's why your moods are like big waves, up and down and up and down...

Yasmine explained her tiredness likewise:

> It's definitely made me tired, it's not the kind of tiredness that I knew.

However, she also said:

> Mind you I've been travelling a lot to the Midlands, these are day trips and make the day very long, maybe it's the stress of my new job.

This allowed for a more interactive account of her experience. Clare on the other hand attributed her low mood entirely to external causes:

> I know why I'm low (cried), I've been to five friends who've given birth in the last four months...

Interestingly, Sheila felt that she had made a mistake in telling her boss at work about her diagnosis:

> He was very nice about it, very understanding, to be honest I couldn't not tell him, how would I explain breaking down and crying at work and all that.

However, he later blamed her menopause, albeit in a sympathetic way, for work-related problems caused by other factors to do with the work environment:

> I came back from leave and found that he'd given the project to a young girl, he

said he didn't think I could cope, but I only didn't finish it before going away because the materials arrived late...

This sparked off a discussion on the varied circumstances in which it might be helpful to disclose aspects of their condition or keep them as private matters.

Relationships and sexuality

Our social world both idealizes the lifelong heterosexual partnership and defines it as the normative lifestyle, particularly for a mature woman. This posed difficulties for most of the group participants and, for Clare in particular, the diagnosis of early menopause had triggered overwhelming anxiety about what was now perceived as an empty life.

She had come to understand that her depression was not just about premature menopause but the gaps in her life that it had highlighted. She arrived at a session having just recovered from flu and said:

I felt really miserable, I was ill, alone in my flat [sobbed]...I just wished there was a man to look after me.

At this point, Ayshe responded with:

Which woman do you know who's looked after by a man rather than looking after men?

The group all laughed. Clare continued:

I'm 33, all my friends have settled down, I've hardly got any single friends any more. They're all preoccupied with their new families, which is the last thing I need from them.

Yasmine did not reveal her recently ended relationship and previous termination but echoed the sadness about not being in a partnership:

something taken for granted when you're in your thirties.

Ayshe was convinced that as a result of early menopause she now looked older and less attractive. She also believed that menopause had slowed down her sex drive. She appeared to have given the subject much thought as she shrugged her shoulders and said in a calm and philosophical tone:

> Well, I don't attract men any more...I feel as if I've gone onto another phase...I
> have a different kind of energy. I also meditate...it has saved me over the years...
> I see things differently now.

Sheila was the only one in the group who had a partner, although the future of their partnership was uncertain. Her diagnosis highlighted a different kind of disappointment. She felt angry towards her partner and their relationship ended for a while:

> I couldn't cope with him not being able to cope...I desperately needed support,
> he wasn't there...When I suggested that we ended the relationship, he didn't
> even bother to try and stop it. I thought, if he doesn't want me, then who's going
> to have me now.

By the end of the group, Sheila and her partner had started talking and she expressed a wish to keep an open mind about their relationship.

Results of evaluation

Attendance

Attendance was 100%.

Verbal feedback

According to the women's accounts in the last and in the individual sessions, the most important aspect of the group appeared to be, for all of them, the positive effect of meeting other women who shared the experience of premature menopause. This effectively put an end to their feelings of isolation and helped to normalize their experience. In the context of the group, early menopause was a mainstream occurrence. All of the women expressed in the group and privately that they would like to exchange telephone numbers and keep in touch.

Future plans

Ayshe identified further psychological help as a future goal and has registered her interest in a new smoking cessation programme.

Clare felt that she needed to widen her social circle, which had been diminishing as a result of old friends moving on to a different lifestyle. While she valued them and wanted to maintain contact, she realized that they now had a different outlook from her and that they would be, at least for a time, preoccupied with young children. By the end of the group she had registered for a diploma course in photography as a step towards her new networking plan. This outcome was the result of the goal planning that she had carried out from session to session, beginning with information gathering about courses.

Sheila wanted to travel. We explored how she could plan for this and she resolved to organize her finances in future with her travel plans in mind. In the meantime, she had adopted a healthier lifestyle and was pleased to have lost 8 lb in weight. When she attended her final (individual) session, however, Sheila informed us that she was pregnant. She described this as a 'major blow'. She said that she had started to feel 'completely adjusted' and 'normal', and that she valued her life just as it was. The pregnancy presented her with a major dilemma.

In the group, Sheila's pregnancy at this time was acknowledged to be very unusual in order not to raise the hopes of other members.

Yasmine was the only one who did not identify a specific plan. She felt that she had needed to process the life changes, that the group had helped her towards it and that she would need to continue the process.

Psychometric measures

Psychometric measures are presented in Table 11.1. The pre-intervention mean CES-D and SWLS scores for these women were remarkably similar to a study conducted two years ago with women who had experienced premature ovarian failure (Liao et al. 1999). On the whole, there appears to be improvement in psychological wellbeing, with four of the six measures changing in the positive direction and two remaining similar.

Table 11.1: Psychometric measures

	Depression		Life satisfaction	
	CES-D (pre)	CES-D (post)	SWLS (pre)	SWLS (post)
Clare	10	2	22	19
Yasmine	36	12	9	22
Ayshe	34	5	8	20
Sheila	15	*	31	*

*Due to the unexpected and difficult circumstances, it was inappropriate to ask this client to complete the post-intervention questionnaires.

Conclusions

This was a brief, focused intervention, which addressed the social and psychological issues in relation to premature menopause. While one of the aims was to increase knowledge and encourage the process of problem solving, it was valued most of all as a forum for the women to reflect on their experience and to explore their personal values about certain existential issues that premature menopause had impacted upon.

The process could also be accomplished on a one-to-one basis. However, the group gave the women the opportunity to come into contact with others who shared similar issues relating to premature menopause. This validates their experience and enables each participant to feel less odd. For these women, as for others whose condition carries a degree of social stigma, the process of sharing, which can only be accomplished in a group situation, is particularly meaningful. While the women had a similar condition, their experiences and perspectives were varied. This helped to shift the constructions each woman held about her problems and helped them to move towards possible solutions. Again, this process is not available on an individual basis.

Informal feedback about the intervention was positive. The women seem to have used the group to identify some of their immediate goals. Their overall wellbeing, as assessed by psychometric measures, appeared to have improved for most of the women. However, the group had certain limitations. Discussions did not go beyond the tentative expression of disagreement to more rigorous debate. Support, facilitation and cooperation are viewed as women's domain. The group process was characterized by cooperation and mutual support and did not reflect the sense of freedom from these limiting views of femininity, to which most of the women professed in discussion. The short duration of the group and its various remits did not enable this process to develop.

While the participants were very distressed at the time of their referral, they were essentially personally resourceful. In the case of Ayshe, who had had chronic difficulties, she had nevertheless achieved a degree of stability in her life, which enabled her to be integrated into the group. Such a group would not have been able to meet the needs of those with more profound and generalized psychological problems, which would be more appropriate for generic psychological services.

The results of this group offer tentative suggestions that brief, structured psychological interventions can help to alleviate distress in the context of premature menopause. However, further work is needed to develop and evaluate a range of psychological interventions and to make them more widely available.

A group experience in Canada

ZELDA ABRAMSON

In 1988, as a social worker in a downtown Toronto hospital, I ran my first information and support group for women experiencing premature menopause. This group proved to be a model for many subsequent groups and training programmes. Although references are made to one group and the participating individuals, the stories and themes are allegorical. I begin by tracing the history of the group's development, which stemmed from an information and support group for menopausal women.

One year after having my second child, I started a new job as a medical social worker, responsible for the gynaecological and surgical wards. Shortly thereafter I was asked to co-lead a menopause group. At 36, I was 15 years younger than the average age of menopause; my colleague was even younger. Although we knew that we were not able to provide support experientially, we nevertheless would be able to provide a supportive venue in which women could share experiences and information.

In times of uncertainty, there is great comfort in information gathering. We feverishly began the task of learning everything there was to know about menopause. This was not an easy undertaking as there were few resources that were not medical. The medical literature, on the other hand, was plentiful and focused on the virtues of HRT, and as a result most medical practices supported widespread use of HRT.

Some of the academic and lay literature on the other hand was critical of medicine's determination to medicalize menopause (McCrea 1983; MacPherson 1981). Women themselves were frightened and confused because of what they had heard of oestrogen's previous record with cancer. Such confusion and scepticism were the motivating factors that underlay women's interest in a group framework. We therefore decided that the format of the group should be structured to provide both information and support. Each week of the four-week sessions, the group focused on a specific topic. Our goal was to enable women to navigate through the difficult choices that had to be made, and then, if needed, that the women continue to meet on their own.

We never needed to advertise these groups. Referrals were either by word of mouth or through women's own resourcefulness. Unlike today, not only were there few books available, but support was difficult to find. As such, these groups were enormously popular, often 15 to 20 women attended each group session. We ran three or four groups a year. Typically the women who attended were white, middle-class and well-educated. The age range varied, with the youngest being 28 and the eldest 56. The majority of women's ages ranged between 45 and 52 years.

In every group, however, there were one or two women whose needs and concerns were not fully addressed. Common to these was their age – under 40 years. These women came to the group knowing that there would be a disjuncture between their concerns as menopausal young women and those of the majority of the group. Caught between two identities, the younger women largely expressed feelings of misfit both in their day-to-day lives and within the menopausal group. Whereas most of their friends were preoccupied with pregnancy, childbirth and babies, they were trying to come to terms with the premature 'ageing' of their reproductive system. Once the focus shifted from the medical to the emotional and the older women talked about children growing up, retirement and ageing parents, the younger women could not relate: to them children leaving home seemed cruel and irrelevant when they themselves were confronting childlessness.

Although these mid-life groups were helpful in terms of providing information and support, the psychosocial issues and concerns confronting younger women were substantively different. We therefore decided to a run a special six-week group for menopausal women under the age of 40 years with emphasis on emotional support. We also felt we had to limit the group to a manageable size to ensure that the needs all of women were met appropriately. Response was greater than anticipated. Initially we had limited the size to 10, but in the end, agreed to 11. Two women decided not to continue and a committed group of nine met weekly.

When planning this group, we felt that the issue of control was central to the lives of women experiencing premature menopause. We knew it was important for this group to steer its course and determine its agenda. The first week therefore focused on introduction and planning. The group decided that their preference was to spend the next two sessions on medical information and the last three sessions on psychosocial matters, such as body image, sexuality/intimate relations, grieving and self-esteem.

The women attending the group were also middle-class, educated and professional. The causes of premature menopause were diverse and ranged from surgical removal of ovaries due to endometriosis or cancer, autoimmune disorders and natural early menopause to medical menopause as a result of radiation or chemotherapy. The group members found the heterogeneous nature (medically) of the group both interesting and helpful in that it was easier to give both information and support. To stand back and objectively self-reflect is a craft that many of us do not have. Women excel, however, in supporting and helping others in a reasonable and thoughtful fashion. So for many of these women the advice and guidance given to the other group members whose conditions were different but ultimately the same, proved invaluable. At the same time as supporting others, these women were able to gain insight and empathy into their own personal circumstances.

Zoe (all names have been changed), who at 30 was diagnosed with cancer, underwent a surgical menopause. She came to the group because she had difficulty coping not only with her disease but with the medical information available to her:

> I had little information about what was to follow in this 'asexual' [no ovaries] state. I was told by [the] oncologist gynecologist that my chronic vaginal yeast infections were due to improper wiping after a bowel movement. 'Hardly', I said. I was told that my vaginal dryness was due to the fact that I was psychologically depressed and it was normal to lose sexual desires at this time. 'Well, you're partly right', I said. I was also told that if I experienced hot flushes to start oestrogen replacement therapy. 'Well I'm not sure that I want that either.'
>
> So, after all this frustration, I decided to take responsibility for my personal health and happiness. I started to read and research information about menopause, oestrogen therapy, sexuality, diet, vitamins, exercise and support groups.
>
> I joined a first of its kind support group [in Toronto]. The support group was set up for women under 40, going through early menopause. I have found the information and emotional sharing invaluable.

The need for medical information cannot be overstated. Many women with premature menopause struggle to manage their physical symptoms. There are both short- and long-term consequences to being menopausal prematurely. The medical community is very clear that for such women HRT is vital. Women with premature menopause have more than a 10-year disadvantage than their cohort vis-à-vis long-term health consequences. Loss of bone mass, for example, accelerates quickly in the years immediately following a woman's last menstrual period. A woman who is menopausal at age 35, by the age of 50 would experience the same bone health problems as a woman of 65 (Lindsay et al. 1978). HRT is advocated for the prevention of osteoporosis and reduced risk of heart disease (Stampfer et al. 1991). However, the question whether long-term oestrogen use may increase a woman's risk for developing breast cancer persists (Colditz et al. 1995; Lancet 1997). The medical community continues to be committed to the benefits of oestrogen and minimizes the significance of the breast cancer risk. Even though heart disease, not breast cancer, is the leading cause of death for women, many women, especially those with pre-existing cancer, remain seriously concerned about using hormones because of the perception of increased risk of breast cancer.

For the women in the group, whether they were experiencing symptoms related to their menopause or whether they were symptom-free, the confusion and controversy surrounding hormone use warranted attention.

> Although I do not have any physical complaints, I continue to be concerned about the benefits and risks of HRT. (I am currently taking oestrogen and progesterone clinically.) I think this concern is complicated because I am a DES daughter (DES was frequently prescribed to women between 1940 and 1960 to prevent miscarriages). Daughters whose mothers took DES are at higher risk for vaginal cancer and other gynaecological disorders. The mothers themselves are now at higher risk for breast cancer, and that in itself holds unknown future health concerns.

> (Laura)

Rachel, on the other hand, started HRT against her better judgement after her uterus and ovaries were removed due to extensive endometriosis:

> I had read and been told endo feeds oestrogen, so I really was concerned about taking medication. It certainly is a lot easier if ovaries can be left in. I did not

want to reactivate endometriosis, so I was concerned about taking oestrogen so soon. The day after surgery I had my first pill.

Three months after experiencing a number of uncomfortable side effects on HRT, her doctor took her off the medication. However, this proved to be difficult in its own right:

> I experienced hot flushes, very minor at first, it was a hot summer so I didn't think a lot about them. They increased in the fall. I now have them less often in [the] day and mostly at night. I have developed carpal tunnel syndrome, with my right hand being worse. I am now coming up to one year of no oestrogen. I have concerns about osteoporosis and the fact that I might be accelerating the process.

> I questioned the need for Provera [synthetic progesterone], as I do not have a uterus, and was told it is prescribed to avoid cysts in the breast. Many of the articles that I read offer different viewpoints on HRT, which makes decisions a little difficult. My dilemma is do I try oestrogen again (low dose)? I was not on a low dose after surgery, which I felt I should have been on.

To address many of the questions surrounding HRT, we invited a physician to the second group session. The physician was asked to present an overview of the pros and cons of HRT, followed by an extensive question-and-answer period. Although we were aware that the physician might only focus on the virtues of HRT, we nevertheless believed that this would be valuable as it would provide more in depth information than that typically available from a five- to 10-minute doctor's appointment. Furthermore, we would be able to 'debrief' the following week – group members would have the opportunity to discuss and evaluate for themselves the biomedical perspective. The intent of the session was not to be critical of medicine but to provide a balance to the medical perspective as it is all too easy in such groups to attack the medical profession:

> My concerns are that of long-term HRT and its consequences. Is it really the answer? Doctors seem to be so ignorant on the subject.

Many women expressed feeling maltreated by the medical profession and had become distrustful of doctors' abilities to be both honest and helpful. Helen's story illustrates this point:

> The HRT failed to restore my sex drive and, once again, the medical experts come up empty. Why didn't they warn me prior to my chemotherapy treatments that loss of sex drive (never mind menopause!) could be one of the long-

term effects? Were they unaware of it or were they afraid I'd refuse chemotherapy? The only place I have ever seen this problem discussed is in Alexander
Solzhenitsyn's novel *The Cancer Ward*, where the protagonist is indeed warned
that chemotherapy for his cancer could terminate his sex life. Ironic, isn't it?
That it's in fiction that we sometimes find the facts to make informed decisions
about our lives. In fiction, the patient has a choice. In fact, I didn't.

Nevertheless, for many others, HRT substantively improved the quality
of their lives. To maintain group cohesion members needed to strike a
balance between a healthy criticism of medicine and at the same time
recognizing its benefits. In so doing, those women who chose HRT
were not alienated from the group, as the central philosophy of the
group was to support women in making informed choices. The actual
decision was less important than that the women felt comfortable with
their choices and believed they were doing what was right for them.

In the third week, the group focused on alternatives to HRT.
Many had already looked into homeopathic and naturopathic remedies and were well-versed in their applications. Such information
sharing was particularly welcomed, especially for those with cancer
who refused HRT.

After three weeks of intensive information sharing, the group was
ready to explore emotional wellbeing. Shame and loss of fertility
were two themes that surfaced repeatedly. More often than not,
shame stems from infertility and for this reason it is difficult to examine them as separate topics. The one woman in the group who
always sported sunglasses personified the depth of shame early
menopausal women may experience. Helen's menopause was kept
secret from everyone, including her husband. Helen was accurate in
her assessment that this shame is taught, not self-imposed: we monitor others' reactions and respond accordingly:

> I went into menopause at the age of 37, a direct result, I believe, of the
> chemotherapy treatment I received for Hodgkin's disease. It was like falling off a
> cliff – into a vacuum. First of all, no one believed I could be menopausal. Not my
> doctor (let's check your thyroid), not the therapist who moderated the
> menopausal support group I tried to get into (you're too young to be
> menopausal!) and certainly not my friends (the last thing they wanted to hear
> was that a contemporary of theirs was showing indisputable signs of ageing), so
> finally even I came to deny the facts.

Defining oneself as menopausal was a struggle, as to be menopausal
implied being 'old'. Claire, who one day while at her mother's house,
realized that she had not taken her hormone pill that day, asked her

mother for one of hers. Her body language squirming, Claire explained:

> We do not share birth control pills with our mothers, neither should we share our hormone replacement pills.

Menopause is frequently associated with negative stereotypes in a culture that emphasizes youth and beauty. Often the language describing menopause is destructive, undermining and anti-woman so that a woman:

> becomes, in the language of misogynists, barren, and to be barren is the quintessential female crime.
>
> (Reitz 1987)

Grief for the loss of fertility was a recurring theme that required frequent revisiting. At times the pain was so intense, it was palpable:

> I feel quite hurt, alienated, and alone in the fact of my age and not being able to bear children which I so dearly wanted.
>
> (Isabel)

The group's success was in its ability to provide a framework where women were not alone in their grief; even a trace of optimism prevailed:

> I have somehow managed to come to terms with the fact that yes, I have gone through menopause, that I am getting older and that in this life at least, I will only have one child (but what a super child he is!). In other words the sight of an older pregnant woman no longer fills me with rage.
>
> (Helen)

The process of healing for many of the women began long before they sought group support. The group was an important next step. Within the group framework, many women were able to work on rebuilding their self-esteem, which had been temporarily lost or mislaid with the onset of menopause:

> Over the last 13 years I have taken what I thought was the easy route, which is ignoring what has happened and the effect it has had on me. Over the last couple of years I have decided to take my head out of the sand and deal with what has happened. I think my major problem has probably been how I view myself. I am starting to develop my self-esteem and realize that I am not less of a woman because I have lost my reproductive organs. I have found little specifically on the

subject of early surgical menopause and, perhaps because I was looking for the 'ultimate solution', I got frustrated and confused with so many opposing views.

(Laura)

For some women, like Zoe, the group was pivotal:

> I have come to recognize and believe that I am a useful, worthy, intelligent and, above all, sexual person. I have come to recognize that I have a lot of living to do. I am better equipped to make intelligent and informed choices about my menopausal symptoms and treatment. I would hope that in the future more support groups evolve in order to fill this need, in that early menopause does exist and has specific concerns, which must be addressed by not only the medical field but by society at large.

Several years later, a number of women continue to meet on an irregular basis. The six-week group provided a structure and support network that could be drawn on as needed.

As with many things in life, my involvement with women experiencing a premature menopause was coincidental. I myself was not menopausal and came to run the group in response to an assessed need. My own personal health status was not kept a secret from the group. It was important for both my colleague and myself not to be viewed as experts, rather facilitators. The expertise came from the participants, those women who experienced menopause.

As a feminist healthcare worker, much of my work focuses on challenging the unequal doctor/patient relationship, and encouraging women to control their healthcare. To do so, I have argued that accessible medical information must be available. This philosophy underpinned the framework of the group. We provided copious amounts of information. More often than not, women left the group more confused than when they started. This, we passionately argued, was a good beginning.

Support group on the net

CATHERINE CORP

> Both the listserv and information packets have enabled me to feel more at ease with my own situation. I am more educated on premature ovarian failure (POF). I have met other women with the same affliction and I don't feel as alone as I did when I was first diagnosed. Most of all, in speaking to the other women through the listserv, I now have hope that one day I may be able to achieve pregnancy through donor egg. This information is most valuable to me. I can't imagine

going through this all alone and the listserv and its members have provided a
much-needed type of support group for women with POF.

(SC, age 28, Ohio, USA, from June 1998 listserv evaluation)

As with many support groups, the Premature Ovarian Failure
Support Group started because of a personal need. When I was
diagnosed with this disorder in 1994 I could find neither information
nor a support system.

I searched books and a database at my county's central library. I
went to book shops. I found little information. Occasionally a book on
menopause mentioned premature menopause but the information was
limited, scary (increased chance of dementia, decreased life span) or
insulting – evidence of POF is rare: it can be mistaken for a pregnancy.

I did a search of organizations (The National Clearinghouse of
Self-help Groups; the Women's Centre in Vienna, Virginia; Resolve
in Washington, DC and New York City; The North American
Menopause Society; and A Friend Indeed). That search failed to
reveal a source of support for women with POF. When I called one
group I was told: 'Just come to our group. We discuss women's
issues.' When I replied that I was looking for something specific on
premature menopause, I was again told that a general group would
suit my needs. I did not think that a general group which would
include women dealing with mid-life menopause, raising children on
their own and/or combining a job and family would help to relieve
my feelings of being 'a freak'. I wanted to talk and see with my own
eyes other women who were experiencing the same thing as I was.

The effect of talking with that organization actually motivated me
to start a group in my area. I had nothing to lose. I made several
phone calls to find a suitable location to meet. A local church agreed
to let us use an adult education classroom one evening per month.
With a small initial outlay I rented a voicemail box, which came with
the option to renew or discontinue after three months. Fortunately
our local newspaper has a weekly guide of support groups provided
free of charge as a community service.

Seven women responded to the first announcement. They ranged
in age from 19 to 43 years. One woman had been diagnosed just a
week before we met; another 12 years earlier. The causes varied and
included autoimmune disorders, genetics, post-chemotherapy for
breast cancer and galactosaemia (an inborn inability to metabolize
the sugar galactose, which, if untreated, accumulates in the blood).

Most women stated that they felt alone, as if they had been hiding a secret. In the words of more than one woman: 'I feel like a freak' – the same words I had used when I was diagnosed – 'no one else has been able to understand how I'm feeling because no one else I know has this disorder'. Finally, we were no longer struggling with this alone. At last we had others with whom we could share our stories. It was a meeting of hope. At that first meeting and in subsequent ones, we discussed how POF affected our relationships with spouses, friends and family; the issue of hormone replacement therapy (HRT); the feeling of being old before our time; the doctor-patient relationship; how to cope during holidays when family with children join us; how to go to that first baby shower for a friend after we have received our diagnosis; and many other topics.

Several of the organizations I had contacted initially sent information about women's health issues and the menopause. I followed up on all the material and eventually saw an article by Dr Larry Nelson at The National Institutes of Health (NIH). He was recruiting women for participation in a POF clinical research study. I live less than 20 miles from NIH. Until the year preceding my diagnosis, I had worked as a paediatric hospice nurse. Many of our patients there were referred from NIH. This was another reason to continue the group and to have it expand. I thought that if I had been so close to our national research centre without knowing about POF research being done there, what were other women doing?

I contacted Dr Nelson and he became an early promoter of our group. Soon after we formed he was interviewed for an article in a women's magazine, *Marie Claire*. At his request our support line number was listed at the end of the article. Over 130 telephone calls from across the country were received by the Washington group.

Three common themes were noted:

- the women felt as if they had aged before their time and that they been dealt a 'double whammy' of infertility and menopause
- there was a paucity of information
- the women wanted to make contact with others in a similar situation.

The need for a national organization seemed clear. Our local group envisioned that such an organization would provide women with strategies to cope with the changes they were experiencing. The purpose was to provide support, information and referrals.

A theoretical framework was adopted as this increased the likelihood that the organization will have long-lasting significance and utility. Yalom's (1980) 'therapeutic or curative factors' provide the basis for the theoretical framework. Four factors were selected for assessment purposes: universality, imparting of information, catharsis and imitative behaviour.

Formal and informal support systems in which women are able to share their feelings and experiences were expanded and new ones developed. We compiled articles that related to POF and distributed them by mail. We gave information over the telephone. And a 'share list' of women with POF was developed. This lists women with POF who want to be in contact with others like themselves. The share list includes names, addresses, telephone numbers and, most recently, e-mail addresses. Confidentiality is vital in maintaining integrity with group members. When women contact us we ask if they would like to be placed on the list. Only those who agree are included and the list goes only to members with POF. We do not share the list with 'others' with whom we communicate. In addition, we started a newsletter, which is published quarterly.

Our group grew very slowly because we are self-sustaining, have not yet established non-profit status and are without funds to expand. One opportunity did present itself. The Endocrine Nurses Society (ENS) put out a call for grant proposals in March 1997 and, as a member of that organization, in June 1997 a grant of $US1500 was awarded. Although not a large sum of money, it did enable us to purchase a computer, install a modem and connect to the Internet. Suddenly, the number of women we could reach had significantly expanded. A web page was created. Originally a one-page introduction with several 'under construction' signs, it greatly expanded over the first year to include a 24-page overview and probably our most successful venture, a listserv. The listserv was created in November 1997 with approximately 60 people, most of them women with POF. In addition, several physicians and nurse researchers interested in POF signed on. Initially most of the subscribers were women from our share list.

On the web site women are free to write about anything pertaining to POF. A monthly issue was attempted but discontinued after a short time. Women exchange information, stories, resources and referrals. On rare occasions, inaccurate information is given out and attempts are swiftly made to correct it. One of the researchers at the NIH periodically analyses the content of the listserv to ensure that correct information is made available. As the group is unmoderated (no one reviews the e-mails before they are sent to our host), 'flames' (one person insulting another on-line) are occasionally posted. This has been the single most distressing aspect in running the listserv because it tends to develop a life of its own. It may not stop at one flame but can develop into several members 'flaming' against others. On two occasions I have had to go on-line and request that the flaming stop.

One component of the ENS grant was an evaluation. A satisfaction survey was to be used to evaluate the effectiveness of the local support groups and the information packets. The surveys were to be distributed by mail but this was altered. The December 1997 newsletter included a questionnaire requesting information on referral sources and asking for ideas in relation to expanding the organization. Only 15% of the members responded. According to direct mail groups this is a number to be proud of. However, we had hoped for higher numbers as this was a highly targeted mailing.

Due to the low response to the December 1997 newsletter, the listserv was used for the evaluation and compiled in June 1998. Analysis showed that over a six-month period the number of subscribers had doubled. At the time of the evaluation there were 121 subscribers, of whom 39 responded. An interesting aspect of doing an evaluation on-line is that there is no way to ensure confidentiality if you request that responses be returned to the group's home e-mail box, as the sender's address is always included. To allow women to respond anonymously and maintain confidentiality, a substitute e-mail box owned by a colleague was given as an alternative. She agreed to receive mail and cut off any identifying headers or footers. Four responses were returned through this second option. Background information and degree of satisfaction on the listserv were elicited.

The age of respondents to the self-report survey ranged from 20 to 41 years, with the majority (25) of responses from women in the 26 to 35 year age bracket. Number of years between diagnosis and current age ranged from one year or less (9 responses) to 10 years or more (5), with most being diagnosed between two or three years (11). The majority (25) had no children. Most (23) had found the listserv through searching on the Internet. In general the listserv was shown to be a valued resource for women. The Internet has increasingly become a way for people to meet one another internationally, and members included women from Australia, England, India and South Africa.

A final comment received from one of the respondents to the list-serv evaluation:

> The listserv is a lifeline, as well as an information line! There are times when I get so depressed and down, and the women on the listserv are really here for me. The information shared both gives me information and gives me questions to ask my doctor...which has improved my treatment. Also, I have to say that I just met one of the women on the listserv. For the first time since we were diagnosed, we were able to have a conversation with someone else struggling with the same diagnosis! I can't even begin to describe how WONDERFUL it was! I realized I had never had a conversation with someone who actually understands! It was really an amazing experience. We talked non-stop, and superfast, for two hours. I hadn't realized how much I needed that. When you think about it, there's almost no experience that so few other people have. Sharing this on-line is unbelievably important, and sharing it in person is basically a miracle.
>
> (AS, aged 38, MA, USA)

Chapter 12
Guidelines for good practice: a biopsychosocial approach

MYRA HUNTER AND DANI SINGER

In this chapter we aim to bring together the key issues raised by the contributors to this book and to suggest points of good practice for those working with women who have experienced premature menopause. Being interdisciplinary, the book brings together the perspectives of health professionals who inevitably have different areas of expertise, points of contact and roles in relation to women who have premature menopause. Some of these roles are highly specific to the particular profession: for example, a consultant in a fertility clinic would be able to offer expert information about his or her treatments. However, other functions and roles are arguably shared by health professionals, such as breaking bad news, offering emotional support and providing clear information. Because of the taboos surrounding premature menopause it is a difficult subject for women to talk about. One of the main pleas by the women whose stories are reported in several chapters was the desire to be listened to and to be taken seriously. It is important, therefore, that all health professionals who may be in contact with women who have experienced premature menopause, no matter how infrequently, do not collude with the taboos and become aware of the range of issues that need to be addressed.

In general, dissatisfactions with healthcare services frequently result from inadequate provision of information, misunderstandings, insensitivity, lack of control over decisions and treatment, and discontinuity of care. There are opportunities for improvement here. This chapter focuses on these and other key issues raised in the preceding chapters, including:

- a biopsychosocial approach to assessment and treatment
- good communication and the provision of information
- acknowledging difference and diversity
- presenting treatment choices and facilitating decision making
- addressing the emotional as well as physical needs.

A biopsychosocial approach to assessment and treatment

A biopsychosocial model is an excellent way of representing the range of influences on an individual's interpretation of a health problem and can be used as a way of thinking about premature menopause and as a framework when communicating with clients (Hunter 1994). Above all, it gives equal value to the biological, psychological, social and cultural factors that shape each person's experience and reactions. For example, the experience of biological changes is inevitably shaped by sociocultural factors, such as beliefs about women's roles and behaviours, and attitudes to ageing and menopause. The model can therefore help us to understand the meaning of premature menopause for a woman in the context of her past and present life (see Figure 12.1).

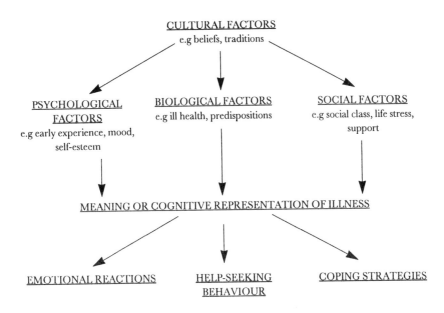

Figure 12.1. A biopsychosocial model

For example, Ms N was suffering from depression six months after a diagnosis of premature menopause. She described herself as an independent person who did not rely on others and who had high standards for herself, particularly at her work as a personal assistant to a barrister. She believed that she should cope with premature menopause herself without any help. By doing so she felt that she was not giving in to the condition and retained her self-esteem, seeing herself as a capable and self-sufficient person. She grew up in a family culture that treated children as 'mini-adults'; this was partly influenced by there being five children and the fact that her mother had health problems throughout her childhood. Ms N learnt to attend to the needs of other family members and derived self-esteem from seeing herself as the strong member of the family. This strategy helped her to become independent and to be successful at work, but was less helpful when she was faced with a more enduring health problem.

When she developed hot flushes and night sweats, Ms N struggled with these symptoms, but became increasingly tired and 'felt a failure'. Unable to maintain her standards at work, she became depressed. In this example we can see how her beliefs about herself, derived from a particular family culture, and her behaviour interacted with physical symptoms to lead to feelings of failure and depression, which also made it difficult for her to seek help. Ms N did, in fact, eventually go to see a counsellor and gradually learnt that having health problems and seeking help need not necessarily be construed as shameful or as failure.

Health psychologists are developing theoretical frameworks to understand people's appraisals and reactions to physical illnesses. One model which is currently being applied to a range of health problems is the Self Regulation Model (Leventhal et al. 1984). The cognitive appraisal of premature menopause can be placed in the centre of the biopsychosocial model; as with Ms N, it was her cognitive appraisal of her illness that influenced her mood and her help-seeking behaviour.

The Self Regulation Model includes five main groups of beliefs that appear to characterize people's appraisals of illness. First, there are a woman's beliefs about what the problem is or its identity (what the bodily symptoms signify), which might include current symptoms, such as hot flushes or tiredness. Second, there are beliefs about causation (what could have caused cessation of menstruation). Beliefs about cause can influence the extent to which the development of the illness makes sense, and also whether or not the person might blame themselves for the illness. These beliefs can affect adjustment to the condition: for example, undue self-blame can lead to depressed mood and a feeling of being unworthy and undeserving of help. Third, is time line, which includes beliefs about duration of symptoms and possible long-term implications of the condition. For example, one person might view premature menopause as a problem only up to the age of 50 when she would then feel 'normal'. Another woman might regard it as a temporary problem that can be dealt with by hormone replacement therapy (HRT). Next, appraisal of the consequences is an important dimension and includes perceptions of the possible impact of premature menopause on health, fertility, relationships and self-esteem. Some of these beliefs are clearly justified, but others may be unduly negative and might be helped to be less catastrophic by talking and testing out assumptions. For example, one woman believed that because she had experienced premature menopause and could not have another child, her husband's feelings for her would change and that the relationship was now at risk. Talking together as a couple with a psychologist enabled her to voice her fears and to be reassured by her partner. Finally, perceptions of control and cure include beliefs about what she can do to help herself, what the medical and non-medical options are for short- and long-term health concerns.

This model provides a useful guideline for the exploration of the woman's appraisal of her condition and is influenced by physical experiences as well as developmental and sociocultural factors. The Self Regulation Model has been used to understand the cognitive appraisal of middle-aged menopause (Hunter & O'Dea 1999) and is being applied to a range of health problems in order to predict emotional reactions, recovery and help-seeking behaviour (see Petrie & Weinman 1997).

From the perspective of a biopsychosocial model, the woman is seen as actively striving to make sense of her situation, developing theories which may change over time, being influenced by information, the views of significant others, experience of other health problems, beliefs about her personal ability to overcome problems or self-efficacy, and attitudes towards illness and seeking help.

In an initial consultation it would be important to ascertain the woman's own beliefs, expectations and level of knowledge about her condition before initiating investigations. As well as providing useful information, this process establishes good rapport and can begin to meet a woman's needs to be listened to and to be taken seriously. If a diagnosis of premature menopause is confirmed, its impact will be shaped by cultural, social and psychological factors, as well as age and life stage. For example, a woman in her thirties who has had three children and has already been sterilized, is likely to evaluate the impact of premature menopause differently, with respect to fertility, from a younger woman who was planning to have children. A recurrent theme throughout this book has been to question assumptions and stereotyped views about women. During an assessment, the health professional might be continually making hypotheses about the likely impact of early menopause for a particular woman based, for example, on information about parity, age, social support and general health. However, these are only hypotheses and they cannot be assumed to be the case unless confirmed by the woman herself. It is more helpful to ask open questions about the woman's own appraisal of the situation at that time, while being aware that other concerns might emerge at later stages. In other words, coming to terms with premature menopause is a process.

Adopting a biopsychosocial approach to treatment means acknowledging the importance of emotional and social support, as well as a range of medical and non-medical treatments. The biopsychosocial model is not fixed but is constantly in a process of change. It can be used to identify possible areas that can be addressed in treatment. For example, the belief that a woman is not attractive if she cannot have children might be challenged, which in turn might lessen the perceived impact of premature menopause on self-esteem. Similarly, people's attitudes to medical treatments may change depending on the severity of symptoms, such as hot flushes, and current life circumstances, such as the demands of working environments (Hunter & O'Dea 1997). In practice then, follow-up and reassessment of needs is an essential part of the healthcare of women diagnosed as having premature menopause. Continuity of care by the same health professional is highly valued. It can be particularly helpful for women to see the same person with whom they shared their initial reactions and concerns. Not only is this continuity perceived as supportive, but it can be useful to monitor change and improvement, for example, in mood over time.

Good communication: the provision of clear and detailed information

One of the most common complaints made by people seeking health care concerns communication – what was and was not said and particularly how information is presented. Knowledge about the cause of the health problem, its prognosis and possible treatments is necessary for people to acquire reasonably accurate expectations, to challenge inaccurate beliefs, to make informed decisions and to prepare psychologically for the future. Most people want to know as much as possible about their health if problems arise. Because premature menopause is often unexpected, many women experience a time of uncertainty before a diagnosis is confirmed. Although it is frequently an upsetting experience, women also expressed relief at discovering what was happening to them (see Chapter 4). The provision of information and support go hand in hand, as support can be communicated by the relationship between the woman and the health professional and the manner in which the information is given and discussed.

Information should be communicated as a two-way process in which the woman's understandings are explored first, such as her thoughts and fears about what may be happening. Women are also likely to have differing expectations of a consultation; for example, some might be looking to gain more information and understanding of the problem and some might want specific treatments, while others might hope for support and counselling. It can be helpful to clarify such expectations in order to meet the person's needs. The health professional needs to listen carefully, being aware of what the woman says and also of her emotional reactions. This is important so that accurate empathy can be communicated by the health professional's mood, non-verbal behaviour and verbal responses, which can reflect back an acknowledgement of the woman's concerns and reactions. Summaries are a useful way to check that your understandings are similar.

There is evidence that some people attending their doctors actively seek out information, called 'monitors', to a greater extent than others who tend not to, called 'blunters' (Miller et al. 1987). Similarly, doctors have been categorized in various ways, for example, according to how much they believe that the patient should be actively involved in the consultation and decision making, and the extent to which they focus on technical and psychosocial aspects of patient care (Grol et al. 1990).

Doctors and patients have also been found to vary in the type of communication they engage in during consultations. In a detailed analysis of the research in this area, Roter (1989) found that for the doctor, information giving happens most frequently (35% of the time), followed by information seeking (22%), positive talk (15%), partnership building (10%), social conversation (6%) and negative talk (1%); for the patient, on the other hand, approximately 50% of the time was spent in information giving and less than 10% in asking questions. If women are to be more involved in the consultation these imbalances may need to be shifted. Health professionals can usefully examine their own beliefs and behaviours during consultations, with the aim of becoming flexible in style, in order to meet patient's needs. Training courses are available to improve communication skills; these are discussed later in this section.

Much work has been carried out to facilitate good communication, notably by Ley and colleagues (Ley 1988). They analysed doctor–patient communication and found that the majority of medical information given is too detailed or complex, and that important information may not be understood or retained by the patient. There is also evidence that doctors and patients might interpret the same information in different ways. Information should be clear and comprehensible; information that is given first and that is emphasized is remembered most. It is important to avoid the use of jargon and unexplained medical terms. Do not give too much information at once. It is best given in clear categories, such as condition, treatment, prognosis and how to cope with the health problem. Information is often available in more than one form, such as leaflets or diagrams. Some patients have found it helpful to tape record an important consultation. Relatives or friends should be invited to assist people with learning difficulties and translators made available to those for whom English is not a first language. There needs to be time for questions and for the person and relatives, if present, to absorb the information. It can be helpful to repeat the information given, to ask the person if they understand and to check if there is anything that they are unclear about.

Even with the best intentions, other factors can impede the process of giving and receiving information. Anxiety, tiredness and ill health can affect concentration and, for many, being in the role of 'patient' undermines their confidence and sense of equality in relationship with the healthcare system. Before a consultation most patients already have some awareness that their problems might be serious and have worries about what they may learn. In one study, recordings were made of doctors giving bad news. Instead of exploring the patients' concerns, doctors tended to immediately give detailed information about the patient's illness and treatment (Maguire 1985). This resulted in the patients still being anxious about their concerns and therefore unable to concentrate properly on the information being imparted.

On receiving unexpected or bad news, shock and distress are common reactions, and some people might express anger. It is helpful to give the patients time to express their feelings, to empathize and to offer support, rather than giving the impression that their feelings are inappropriate. It might be useful to find a place where the person can be alone with a friend or relative for a while to absorb the information before returning to discuss the implications of the news. Anger can be harder to deal with. If it is in reaction to a loss or a diagnosis, this should not be taken personally by the health professional, but if a mistake has been made, then an apology is helpful, along with attempts to prevent this happening again. Being defensive in these situations can exacerbate the distress and anger. Maria, for example, on learning that she had a premature menopause, was upset and angry at her gynaecologist when the news was initially broken. The doctor said that he understood that she was upset, but it was only after further exploration that he discovered that she had been trying to find out what was wrong with her for between two and three years. He empathized with her frustration; she was in fact not angry with him but that the 'vague symptoms' she had been reporting to her GP had not been recognized as premature menopause. It is important not to try to identify blame but to listen and to take the issue seriously.

At the end of the interview it can be useful to let the person know how much time is left, to summarize the information and the implications discussed, and to arrange a follow-up appointment so that further questions can be answered. Health professionals need time to process the giving of bad news as well. That is why some preparation should be given to such consultations, for example, giving adequate time and some thought to the person's expectations and possible concerns. In addition, after a distressing session the health professional should allow some time to reflect on the interview and his or her own feelings.

Feelings of rejection or inadequacy may be a result of the individual's anger or distress and the inability of health professionals to remove this distress. On the other hand, to contain and listen to these feelings is in itself therapeutic and is an example to the woman that her feelings are valid, that she is being taken seriously and that it is acceptable to have such feelings. However, health professionals are more likely to explore a woman's emotional reactions if they feel that they will be supported both practically and emotionally by their colleagues. It can be helpful to foster an environment in which it is acceptable to have supervision and an opportunity to debrief or receive feedback about a difficult situation. Team case discussions, during which it is acknowledged that all professionals, regardless of experience, can find giving bad news difficult and emotionally upsetting, can be a useful forum. Moreover, the health worker needs to know who to refer on to and seek advice from, such as counselling, psychology or psychiatric services, if they feel that their skills are not adequate to meet the individual's future needs.

Increased attention is now being given to communication skills in medical and nurse training. For example, students can be taught active listening, empathy, use of open-ended questioning, use of eye contact, summarizing and the skills of developing a shared understanding of the person's problem. These skills can be taught in different ways, but the most successful tend to employ active learning and simulated role plays as well as real patient interviews. Constructive feedback is given and video recordings are increasingly being used. Courses for qualified staff are also available, using tape- and video-recorded role plays with constructive feedback; these can provide an excellent method of improving communication skills (see Fallowfield 1993). Improving communication skills is an important aspect of the biopsychosocial approach, because good communication skills facilitate an individual's involvement in the healthcare process, help the health professional to address both the physical and emotional needs of the person, reduce anxiety, and facilitate information giving and recall, as well as satisfaction and adherence to treatments.

Acknowledging difference and diversity

As outlined above, communication needs to be clear and information should be given in a sensitive way. However, the health professional also needs to be aware of the differences between women in their expectations and needs and to acknowledge that women seeking help may have different value systems and social and cultural backgrounds form themselves. Agnes Marfo has described in Chapter 6 how beliefs and practices vary between cultures and between ethnic groups living in the UK.

Women seeking help for problems relating to premature menopause may vary along the following dimensions: race, culture, gender, sexual identity, age, parity, marital status, socioeconomic status, beliefs about the menopause, and beliefs about doctors and medical treatments. Health professionals will also have varied backgrounds and beliefs. Because premature menopause evokes beliefs and assumptions about gender and reproduction, health professionals need to be aware of their own attitudes and beliefs so that these do not overly interfere with their relationships with patients and the advice they offer. For example, if a woman has a career it should not be assumed that she will be less distressed by infertility. If a woman is from a particular culture she may not conform to stereotypic views about that culture. Obviously, it is also important not to assume that all women are heterosexual. Some women have strong views about medication and the extent to which they wish to use it. Others may not feel strongly about fertility but have concerns and fears about future health. Doctors vary too in their values and beliefs about medication and non-medical approaches. For example, some doctors advocate HRT use for preventative health more strongly than others.

There is not one prescription for dealing with diversity apart from becoming aware of, questioning and resisting one's own assumptions and stereotyped beliefs about other people in healthcare settings. By exploring women's expectations and beliefs using open questions the scene is being set for acceptance of differences. You can check with the person whether an understanding or belief is something that is shared by her family, or friends or her culture. For example, Daljeet told her doctor that her parents did not want her to discuss her premature menopause with anyone else; they felt ashamed and worried that no one would want to marry her if they found out. Daljeet felt that this was making it harder to deal with because she wanted to tell her two close friends but also felt that loyalty to her parents was very important. The doctor in this situation acknowledged that it must have been difficult for her to talk to him and asked her more about whether she thought her parents' reactions were common in other families in her culture or whether she felt that they were more worried than others might be. It transpired that although she felt that to keep silent was consistent with her cultural beliefs and practices, she thought that her parents were overprotective towards her and overly worried about her future. This led to Daljeet planning to go back and discuss her views about her future with her parents; she decided to reassure them but also let them know what would be helpful to her, i.e. confiding in two other women that she could trust.

The framework of the biopsychosocial model, which takes account of the influence of culture and social situation upon lifestyle and health beliefs, can be a useful way of acknowledging differences during a consultation. Some health professionals find it helpful to have a diagram of the model to use with each individual to discuss the factors that may be particularly relevant for her (see Hunter 1994).

Presenting treatment choices and facilitating decision making

Effective communication is also crucial in situations where people are required to make important decisions relating to their health. Women who have received a diagnosis of premature menopause are confronted with many questions and decisions. For example, whether to have HRT, if so what form to take and for how long, whether to pursue fertility treatment or consider adoption or not, whether to have counselling, seek peer support or use non-medical approaches. In these situations it is not only information or extent of knowledge that is important, but also the woman's beliefs, expectations and values that need to be taken into account.

It helps in these situations to let the person know that there are choices even though the health professional might feel strongly that the weight of evidence is in favour of a particular course of action. It is the responsibility of the health professional to draw attention to choices that the woman might not be aware of and then to present the information about the pros and cons of these from the medical perspective. This includes the evidence about their efficacy, contraindications, possible side effects and longer-terms health risks. In areas where the evidence is unclear or more research is needed, this should be acknowledged. Most decisions involve making a choice about two or more options and weighing the balance between outcomes, each having their advantages and disadvantages. When facing a difficult decision mixed feelings are to be expected; there is likely to be uncertainty, whatever the decision. For example, Mr and Mrs F were contemplating a decision whether to pursue egg donation or to approach an adoption society. Eventually they decided to try for egg donation but to do this for a period of two years, which would leave them enough time to work towards adopting a child should egg donation be unsuccessful. This decision took them several months to make and each spoke to medical experts, a fertility counsellor, friends and family. The process involved them putting forward their preferences individually and then negotiating a shared decision. Mrs F was keener on the egg donation option, while Mr F was initially concerned about his wife having to endure further physical trauma and preferred adoption. The solution they agreed on included an important time element that enabled them to explore both options sequentially.

When facilitating decision making, it is important to acknowledge that the woman has knowledge and opinions that she brings to the situation. She may arrive at the consultation, be presented with information, then re-evaluate her initial position. It is helpful to explore her views about treatments, for example, some people do not like to take medication for a long period of time, while others do not like to take tablets daily because they are reminded of the health problem. The way that information is presented can influence decision making. In one study of consultations in which women were asked to consider the risks (miscarriage) and benefits (identifying an abnormality) of having amniocentesis, doctors' use of words like 'high' or 'moderate', paired with the percentage risk, significantly influenced women's choices (see Marteau 1994). For example, a 30% risk of miscarriage could arguably be considered to be relatively low or quite high. A useful strategy is to present the percentages, if relevant, first and then to discuss what they mean to the woman and doctor.

In the past 10 years much research has been focused on the decision of whether or not to take HRT for women facing mid-life menopause. The issues include having relevant information, consideration of the potential risks and benefits, an awareness of her own health history and her personal risks resulting from genetic and lifestyle factors, and her preferences. In a study examining women's attitudes to HRT, Rothert (1991) found that generally women desired more information about the menopause and HRT, but that their needs for information were not being met. The potential risks and benefits of HRT have been outlined in Chapters 7 and 8.

There is evidence to suggest that middle-aged women tend to base decisions on their experience of current symptoms, such as hot flushes and night sweats, while doctors and health professionals tend to emphasize the longer-term preventative benefits of HRT (Ferguson et al. 1989). This difference in perspectives can lead to dissatisfaction with consultations and low adherence rates (Hibbard & Hampson 1993). In a recent qualitative study of decision making about HRT, three main areas were mentioned by women when they described the reasons for or against having hormonal therapy. The first was the severity of hot flushes and night sweats, the second was their doctors' views and advice, and the third their beliefs about taking hormone treatment for what they saw as a 'natural' process. Many felt that it was better to avoid medication if possible; they believed that it was not 'natural' to take medication when there were no signs of illness. However, if vasomotor symptoms were troublesome, then the menopause could be seen as more of an illness and it was felt to be reasonable to have treatment. Other reasons included a family history of osteoporosis and practical reasons, for example, an important social event for one woman made it more important for her to have relief from hot flushes at that particular time (Hunter et al. 1997).

For women dealing with premature menopause the issue of prevention is more important, since HRT is strongly recommended for the prevention of osteoporosis especially for women having premature menopause. Concerns about long-term use of medication and beliefs about hormonal therapies should be taken seriously and discussed. Women will need balanced information and the opportunity to discuss the complex issues involved, such as the relative costs and benefits for them, and to air concerns about what is known about the long-term effects of HRT. The importance of information is generally recognized, but the need for women to make decisions that are consistent with their own beliefs and lifestyles should also be recognized. Research is currently being undertaken to investigate types of interventions that can facilitate decision making relating to HRT use. For example, Hampson and Hibbard (1996) advocate an educative approach to empower women to overcome barriers to communication, such as lack of information and stigma of the menopause, differing agendas and power relationships between women and health professionals. Leaflets, lectures and videos have also been used, and in one study, a decision support intervention aims to actively involve women in assessing their beliefs and personal health risks (Rothert et al. 1994). Much of this work has been carried out with middle-aged women; further work is needed to explore treatment decisions for younger women facing menopause. Nevertheless, the need for information and discussion, with active involvement of the woman, giving consideration to her individual needs and values, would seem to be important regardless of the age of menopause.

Finally, if decision making is particularly difficult for someone, it might be because she is too distressed to think clearly about the future implications of a decision because it is too difficult to think ahead. There is always more time. Decisions should not be rushed. Similarly, if the issues are morally or ethically complex or if the health professional is not familiar with the literature on a particular choice, it is better to be honest and refer the person to someone who has more specialist information or expertise, for example to a fertility clinic, a menopause clinic, an appropriate self-help organization or for a second opinion.

Addressing the emotional as well as physical needs

The importance of good communication and detailed medical assessment for women who might have premature menopause has been emphasized in chapters throughout this book. For example, a comprehensive medical history is essential and relevant investigations need to be discussed with clear explanations. Alternative diagnoses should be considered before making a final diagnosis and this is then to be communicated with sensitivity, giving time for the person to process the information to some extent and to ask questions. Further appointments are useful to provide a forum for further discussion and questioning, as well as continuing to address medical issues. Commonly questions include those pertaining to cause/s, consequences (both short- and long-term), prognosis and possible treatments. These are broadly the areas covered by the Self Regulation Model (Leventhal et al. 1984) and reflect the kinds of thoughts and concerns that are common reactions to physical illness. Following the initial diagnosis and immediate medical attention, many women report that their physical needs have been met but their emotional needs have not. Because of the stigma of infertility and menopause, and other people's reactions of surprise and curiosity, it can often be difficult for a woman to initiate seeking help for her emotional reactions to premature menopause.

Before describing the kinds of approaches that can address the emotional needs of women experiencing premature menopause, we will describe the process of adjustment which is applicable to any negative life event. As mentioned earlier in this chapter, women's appraisals of a diagnosis of premature menopause are not static; they continue to change through a process during which a variety of cognitive interpretations and emotional reactions occur. In her work on terminal illness, Kubler-Ross (1970) describes stages of adjustment. These stages are akin to reactions following bereavement and any significant loss. They include:

- shock, numbness, or disbelief on initially hearing the diagnosis. This has been called the period of denial when the bad news seems too overwhelming to be fully absorbed
- distress as the reality of the situation is faced. Strong feelings of anxiety, anger, thoughts such as 'if only I had done this or that I might have prevented this...'
- depression and despair. This stage is the grieving sad stage during which the loss is emotionally processed
- gradual adjustment and acceptance of the situation; the significance of the loss or illness is incorporated into the person's perceptions of themselves and their future plans.

There is, however, a substantial variation between people in their experience of this adjustment process. Some show acceptance soon after the diagnosis, while others might find that one stage predominates, for example anger or denial. People can also oscillate between stages, and the time each stage lasts is extremely variable. While the empirical evidence for a stage theory of adjustment is not very strong (Silver & Wortman 1991), most researchers agree that there is a process of emotional and cognitive processing that is necessary and that this takes time (Rachman 1980). Horovitz (1986), one of the leading cognitive psychologists in the field, describes how a major life event or loss challenges a person's basic assumptions about the world, themselves and the future. In order to come to terms with this the person has to readjust certain beliefs and assumptions, such as 'I am a healthy person', 'If I behave in a certain way I can avoid bad things from happening to me', in the light of the new information.

In this context, strong emotional reactions to a diagnosis of premature menopause should be expected; they may not be expressed at the time because of the initial shock, but they are part of the process and it can be helpful to acknowledge them by inquiring about a woman's feelings at each consultation. For many people extreme emotional reactions are frightening in themselves and it can be reassuring for them to know that the health professional recognizes that these are normal and common reactions. Health professionals are often asked whether certain reactions are 'normal'.

It would be fair to say that following a major loss a wide range of reactions and feelings are experienced. It is often their duration and the extent to which they interfere with life in the longer term that might raise questions about whether psychological help would be indicated. For example, in most cases a supportive relationship in which the person can talk openly about their thoughts and feelings can be helpful in facilitating adjustment. The other person might be a friend, partner or someone else who has had a similar experience. However, if over time there is no gradual lessening of distress, or if the person's reactions are having a major impact on their ability to function, then additional help may be suggested.

Certain types of beliefs may be associated with prolonged distress, such as excessive guilt or self-blame, and beliefs which impede emotional expression, such as 'It is weak to cry' or 'I should not be upset because it will upset my family' can make it difficult to process the emotional reactions to the diagnosis. Cognitive therapy would be an appropriate treatment in these situations; with the therapist, usually a clinical psychologist, the woman could examine the implications of these beliefs and explore other alternatives.

Cognitive therapy has been applied to other medical problems; for example, it has been found to be more effective than counselling in patients adjusting to a diagnosis of cancer (Moorey & Greer 1989). Cognitive behavioural therapy for anxiety and depression would similarly focus on cognitions and behavioural strategies that might facilitate adjustment, such as setting goals to engage in activities that provide self-esteem, and helping a person to counter overly self-critical thoughts, such as 'If I am infertile I am unlovable', 'I have aged overnight'. For a detailed discussion of cognitive behavioural approaches, see Salkovskis (1996) and Hawton et al. (1989).

Another group of people who might need more support and counselling might be those who lack a confidante or close relationship, or who have a partner or family member who is actively unsupportive. Inquiring about available social support can be useful. One woman felt that she would have been able to deal with her own feelings herself, but because her partner reacted so negatively to the situation she found herself supporting him, thereby impeding her ability to process her own feelings. A strategy that can work in the short term but may be less helpful in the longer term is to become very busy and distract oneself by work or other activities. For some people this is a common coping strategy, but for others it may be thrust upon them. For example, if another major life event happens at around the same time it can be difficult to grieve two losses. A loss of a family member, a child's illness or a redundancy can lead to a focus away from the processing of premature menopause. In these situations women need to be encouraged to take time to think and look after themselves, rather than others, in order to come to terms with what has happened. Sometimes practical advice such as this is helpful in itself; giving people permission to concentrate on themselves and to look after themselves both physically and emotionally can be healing and can counter low self-esteem and negative self-critical thoughts.

There is a need to strike a balance between the exploration of the meaning of the losses that premature menopause potentially entails, and valuing the individual's coping skills and positive competencies. Women who actively seek to be involved in dealing with the situation may fare better psychologically than those who try to avoid the issue altogether. However, embarking too quickly on 'solutions', such as fertility treatments, before working through the feelings of loss may not be the best course of action. Issues of self-esteem need to be addressed, even if parenthood is achieved. Fertility treatment can involve considerable stress and in these situations supportive counselling can be helpful. Self-esteem, the loss of which can lead to depression, is closely connected to sociocultural beliefs about what a woman should be and do. 'Cognitive mediation' between external social attitudes and an individual's self-image, that is addressing the thoughts that intervene between events and emotional responses to infertility, may be particularly useful in this context (see Hunt & Monach 1997).

For some women, a diagnosis of premature menopause may evoke earlier unresolved losses or early life experiences as well as being a 'situational crisis', that is a sudden disruption of current expectations and life plans. While it is important to acknowledge the physiological basis of the difficulties encountered, and the person's cognitive and emotional responses to them, it may also be helpful for some women to look further into their particular emotional responses to premature menopause. Some may feel strongly that their bodies have betrayed them and react by overeating or neglecting themselves (Hendricks 1985). As described in Chapter 5, the inability to produce a child may represent a failure to achieve one of life's traditional milestones, 'generativity' (Erikson 1965), and a wound to self-esteem. A safe place and an opportunity to ventilate and understand reactions to hidden, and often socially unacceptable, losses can be provided in counselling and/or psychotherapy settings.

Damaged self-worth may result from experiencing a broad range of emotions, such as guilt, shame, jealousy, anger and helplessness. These might be unexpressed or directed outwardly towards family, friends or health professionals. These feelings are often difficult to share. In a counselling relationship such feelings can be accepted and understood, and for many women with premature menopause eventually alternative life goals and meanings are found. Health professionals can also help women to break through the isolation of premature menopause by encouraging them to talk to those they trust and from whom they are likely to derive support.

Support groups can be a valuable source of information and support for women dealing with premature menopause, as described in Chapter 11. As well as processing the emotional reactions to the diagnosis, women also have to deal with physical changes, such as hot flushes and night sweats. Although many choose to have HRT to relieve these short-term symptoms as well as possible long-term health problems, such as osteoporosis and cardiovascular problems, some prefer to use non-medical approaches. These have been outlined in detail in Chapter 8. An additional treatment developed for hot flushes includes relaxation therapy, information, and monitoring of hot flushes and night sweats. Precipitators of the symptoms are recognized and modified when possible and women are taught general stress management. This treatment is a form of cognitive-behaviour therapy and has been shown to be effective in reducing menopausal hot flushes (Hunter & Liao 1996).

Other specific forms of psychological interventions might be appropriate for women with particular needs. For example, adjustment to premature menopause might in the long term be more difficult for people who have pre-existing problems with relationships, low self-esteem or emotional problems. Counselling, cognitive-behaviour therapy or psychotherapy can be helpful in providing support, identification of thoughts and feelings, and an opportunity to test out thoughts and assumptions about oneself and others. Some general practices have counsellors and clinical psychologists, and many local hospitals have clinical psychology and psychotherapy departments. Psychological therapy is also available privately; it is important to advise patients to seek a therapist with recognized qualifications. See Resources p. 275 for relevant organizations.

We hope that in this and the preceding chapters the point has been made that it is the counselling skills of all health professionals who help women with premature menopause that are crucial. The way in which the news is broken, the initial emotional support given, and the acknowledgement of its potentially difficult and varied impact can make a positive difference to how women adjust to this often unexpected life event.

References

Abdalla HI, Baber R, Kirkland A, Leonard T, Power M, Studd JWW (1990) A report on 100 cycles of oocyte donation: factors affecting the outcome. Human Reproduction 5: 1018.

Abdalla HI, Billett A, Kan AKS, Baig S, Wren M, Korea L, Studd JWW (1998) Obstetric outcome in 232 ovum donation pregnancies. British Journal of Obstetrics and Gynaecology 105: 332-7.

Abdalla HI, Leonard T (1988) Cryopreserved zygote intrafallopian transfer for anonymous oocyte donation. Lancet 1: 835.

Abdalla HI, McKay Hart D, Lindsay R, Leggate I, Hooke A (1985) Prevention of Bone Mineral Loss in Postmenopausal Women by Norethisterone. Obstetrics and Gynecology 66(6): 789-92.

Abdalla HI, Wren ME, Thomas A, Korea L (1997) Age of the uterus does not affect pregnancy or implantation rates; a study of egg donation in women of different ages sharing oocytes from the same donor. Human Reproduction 12: 827-9.

Abernethy K (1997a) Dealing with the devastating effects of early menopause. Community Nurse 3(2): 48-9.

Abernethy K (1997b) The Menopause and HRT. London: Baillière Tindall.

Adlercreutz H, Hulthen K, Tikkanen M J (1998) Phytoestrogens in menopause (Abstract). International Journal of Fertility and Women's Medicine 43(4): 206.

Ahuja KK, Mostyn BJ, Simons EG (1997) Egg sharing and egg donation: attitudes of British donors and recipients. Human Reproduction 12: 2845-52.

Ahuja KK, Simons EG, Fiamanya W, Dalton M, Armar NA, Kirkpatrick P, Sharp S, Arian-Schad M, Seaton A, Watters AJ (1996) Egg sharing in assisted conception: ethical and practical considerations. Human Reproduction 11: 1126-31.

Ain KB, Mori Y, Refetoff S (1987) Reduced clearance rate of thyroxine-binding globulin (TBG) with increased sialylation: a medium for estrogen-induced elevation of serum TBG concentration. Journal of Clinical Endocrinology and Metabolism 65(40): 689-96.

Aittomaki K (1994) The genetics of XX gonadal dysgenesis. American Journal of Human Genetics 54: 844-51.

Aittomaki K, Herva U-H, Juntunen K, Ylostalo P, Hovatta O, de la Chapelle A (1996) Clinical features of primary ovarian failure caused by a point mutation in the follicle-stimulating hormone receptor gene. Journal of Clinical Endocrinology and Metabolism 81: 3722-6.

Aittomaki K, Lucena JLD, Pakarinen P, Sistonen P, Tapanainen J, Gromoll J, Kaskikari R, Sankila E-M, Lehvaslaiho H, Engel AR, Neischlag E, Huhtaniemi I, de la Chapelle A (1995) Mutation in the follicle-stimulating hormone receptor gene causes hereditary hypergonadotropic ovarian failure. Cell 82: 959-68.

American Fertility Society, Society for Assisted Reproductive Technology (1994) Assisted reproductive technology in the United States and Canada: 1992 results generated from American Fertility Society/Society for Assisted Reproductive Technology Registry. Fertility and Sterility 62:1121-8.

Amundson DW, Diers CJ (1970) The age of the menopause in classical Greece and Rome. Human Biology 42:79-86.

Amundson DW, Diers CJ (1973) The age of the menopause in medieval Europe. Human Biology 45: 605-12.

Anasti JN (1998) Premature ovarian failure: an update. Fertility and Sterility 70(1): 1-15.

Anasti JN, Kalantaridou SN, Kimzey LM, Defensor RA, Nelson LM (1998) Bone loss in young women with karyotypically normal spontaneous premature ovarian failure. Obstetrics and Gynecology 1: 12-15.

Anderson DC (1974) Sex-hormone-binding globulin. Clinical Endocrinology 3: 69-96.

Andrews B, Brown GW (1995) Stability and change in low self-esteem: the role of psychosocial factors. Psychological Medicine 25: 23-31.

Andrews LV (1993) Women at the Edge of Two Worlds. New York: Harper Collins.

Arias AR (1950) La menopausia precoz y su tratamento hormonal. Revista Medica de Chile 78: 373.

Arif S, Vallian S, Farazneh F, Zanone M, James SL, Pietropaolo M, Hettiarachichi S, Vergani D, Conway GS, Peakman M (1996) Identification of 3Beta-hydroxysteroid dehydrogenase as novel target of steroid-producing cell autoantibodies: association of autoantibodies with endocrine autoimmune disease. Journal of Clinical Endocrinology and Metabolism 81(12): 4438-45.

Aristotle (ca 350 BC) Historia Animalium, Book VII (trans R Cresswell). London: George Bell and Sons (1897). Quoted in Ginsburg J (1991) What determines the age at the menopause? British Medical Journal 302: 1288-9.

Asch RH, Balmaceda JP, Ord T, Borrero C, Cefalu E, Gastaldi C et al. (1988) Oocyte donation and gamete intra fallopian transfer in premature ovarian failure. Fertility and Sterility 49: 263.

Asch RH, Ellsworth LR, Balmaceda JP, Wong PC (1984) Pregnancy after translaparoscopic gamete intrafallopian transfer. Lancet 2: 1034-5.

Ashby TA (1894) The influence of minor forms of ovarian and tubal disease in the causation of sterility. Transactions of the American Gynecological Society 19: 260-71.

Aubard Y, Teissier MP, Grandjean MH et al. (1997) Early menopause. Journal du Gynecologie Obstetrique et Biologie de la Reproduction 26: 231-7

Avis NE, Kaufert PA, Lock M, McKinlay SM, Vass K. (1993) The evolution of menopausal symptoms. In Burger HG (ed) The Menopause. London: Baillière Tindall.

Avis NE, McKinlay SMA (1991) A longitudinal analysis of women's attitudes towards the menopause: results from the Massachusetts women's health study. Maturitas 3: 65-79.

Aziz R (1997) Feminism and the challenge of racism: deviance or difference? In Safia Mirza H (ed) Black British Feminism: a reader. London: Routledge.

Baber R, Abdalla HI, Studd J (1991) The premature menopause. In Studd J (ed) Progress in Obstetrics and Gynaecolgy, vol 9. London: Churchill Livingstone, pp 209-26.

Bagur AC, Mautalen CA (1992) Risk for developing osteoporosis in untreated premature menopause. Calcified Tissue International 51(1): 4-7.

Bakare-Yusuf B (1997) Raregrooves and raregroovers: a matter of taste, difference and identity. In Safia Mirza H (ed) Black British Feminism: a reader. London: Routledge.

Baker TG (1963) A quantitative and cytological study of germ cells in human ovaries. Proceedings of the Royal Society of London 158: 417-33.

Balen AH, Jacobs HS (1997) Infertility in Practice. Edinburgh: Churchill Livingstone.

Barlow DH (1996) Premature ovarian failure. Ballière's Clinical Obstetrics and Gynaecology 10(3): 361-84.

Bartholet E (1993) Family Bonds. Boston: Houghton Mifflin.

Bates A, Howard PJ (1990) Distal long arm deletions of the X chromosome and ovarian failure. Journal of Medical Genetics 27: 722-3.

Benedek T (1948) Menopause as a developmental phase in psychoanalytic investigations. New York: Quadrangle, pp 322-49.

Benedek T (1950) Climacterium: a developmental phase. Psychoanalytic Quarterly 19: 1-27.

Bennett C (1996) The clock in the waiting womb. The Guardian 20 Feb: 2-3.

Beral V (1997) Breast cancer and hormone replacement therapy: collaborative re-analysis of data from 51 epidemiological studies of 52,705 women with breast cancer and 108,411 women without breast cancer. Collaborative Group on Hormonal Factors in Breast Cancer. Lancet 349: 1047-59.

Beresford SAA, Weiss NS, Voigt LF, McKnight B (1997) Risk of endometrial cancer in relation to use of oestrogen combined with cyclic progestagen therapy in postmenopausal women. Lancet 349: 458-69.

Bergkvist L, Adami H-G, Persson I, Bergstrom R, Krusemo UB (1989) Prognosis after breast cancer diagnosis in women exposed to estrogen and estrogen-progestogen replacement therapy. American Journal of Epidemiology 130: 221-8.

Bertrand-Servais M, Letur-Konirsch H, Raoul-Duval A, Frydman R (1993) Psychological considerations of anonymous oocyte donation. Human Reproduction 8(6): 874-9.

Beyenne Y (1986) Cultural significance and physiological manifestations of the menopause: a biocultural analysis. Culture, Medicine and Psychiatry 10: 47-71.

Billig H, Chun SY, Eisenhaur K, Hsueh J (1996) Gonadal cell apoptosis: hormone-regulated cell demise. Human Reproduction Update 2(2): 103-17.

Bines J, Oleske DM, Cobleigh MA (1996) Ovarian function in premenopausal women treated with adjuvant chemotherapy for breast cancer. Journal of Clinical Oncology 14(5): 1718-29.

Birge JB (1996) Is there a role for estrogen replacement therapy in the prevention and treatment of dementia? Journal of the American Geriatrics Society 44: 865-70.

Bjoro K (1966) Amenorrhea: a study with particular attention to the problems of ovarian failure. Acta Obstetrica et Gynecologica Scandinavica 45 (suppl 1): 69.

Blumenfeld Z, Golan D, Halachmi S, Makler A, Peretz BA, Brandes JM, Shmuel Z (1993) Premature ovarian failure – the prognostic application of auoimmunity on conception after ovulation induction. Fertility and Sterility 59: 750-5.

Blyth E (1995) Infertility and Assisted Conception: practice issues for counsellors. Birmingham: British Association of Social Workers Publications.

Blyth E (1998) Secrecy and anonymity in donor-assisted conception: a view from a family through adoption. In Blyth E, Crawshaw M, Speirs J (eds) Truth and the Child 10

Years On: information exchange in donor-assisted conception. Birmingham: British Association of Social Workers Publications.

BMA (1996) Changing Conceptions of Motherhood: the practice of surrogacy in Britain. London: BMA.

BMA (1993) Complementary Therapies: A consumer checklist. London: BMA.

Bollas C (1995) Cracking Up. London: Routledge.

Borini A, Bianchi L, Violini F, Maccolini A, Cattoli M, Flamigni C (1996) Oocyte donation program: pregnancy and implantation rates in women of different ages sharing oocytes from single donor. Fertility and Sterility 65: 94-7.

Bosley S, Ward D (1999) Menopause Reversal Proclaimed The Guardian (News) September 24th p3.

Boston Collaborative Drug Surveillance Program (1974) Surgically confirmed gallbladder disease, venous thromboembolism, and breast tumours in relation to postmenopausal estrogen therapy. New England Journal of Medicine 290: 15-19.

Boulet M, Lehert PH, Riphagen FE (1985) The menopause viewed in relation to other life events – a study performed in Belgium. Maturitas 10: 333-42.

Bowles C (1986) Measure of attitude towards menopause using the semantic differential model. Nursing Research 35(2): 81-5.

Bridges W (1980) Transitions: making sense of life's changes. Don Mills, Ontario: Addison-Wesley.

British Hyperlipidaemia Association (1998) HRT in Hyperlipidaemic Post Menopausal Women (Advice Sheet 1)

Brodzinsky D, Schecter M (eds) (1990) The Psychology of Adoption. Oxford: Oxford University Press.

Bromwich P (1990) Oocyte donation. British Medical Journal 300: 1671-2.

Bronner F (1994) Calcium and osteoporosis. American Journal of Clinical Nutrition. 60(6): 831-6.

Burger H, Davis S (1998) Should women be treated with testosterone? Clinical Endocrinology 49: 159-60.

Burger HG (1996) The menopausal transition. Baillières Clinical Obstetrics and Gynaecology 10: 347-59.

Busacca M, Fusi FM, Brigante C, Doldi N, Vignali M (1996) Success in inducing ovulation in a case of premature ovarian failure using growth-releasing hormone. Gynecological Endocrinology 10(4): 277-9.

Byrne J, Fears TR, Gail MH, Pee D, Connelly RR, Austin DF, Homes GG, Homes FF, Latorette HB, Meigs JW et al. (1992) American Journal of Obstetrics and Gynaecology 166(3): 788-93.

Calman K, Moores Y (1998) Clinical examination of the breast. Department of Health, Professional Letter.

Cameron IT, O'Shea FC, Rolland JM (1988) Occult ovarian failure: a syndrome of infertility, regular menses, and elevated follicle-stimulating hormone concentrations. Journal of Clinical Endocrinology and Metabolism 67: 1190-4.

Campbell S, Whitehead MI (1977) Oestrogen Therapy and the Menopausal Syndrome. Clinics in Obstetrics and Gynaecology 4. London and Philadelphia: WB Saunders, pp 31-47.

Campioni M (1997) Revolting women: women in revolt. In Komesaroff P, Rothfield P, Daly J (eds) Reinterpreting Menopause: cultural and philosophical issues. New York: Routledge.

Cano F, Simon C, Remohi J et al. (1995) Effect of aging on the female reproductive system: evidence for a role of uterine senescence in the decline in female fecundity. Fertility and Sterility 64: 584-9.

Case records of the Massachusetts General Hospital (1986) Case 46-1986. A 26-year-old woman with secondary amenorrhoea. New England Journal of Medicine 315: 1336-43.

Cassou B, Derriennic F, Monfort C, Dell'Accio P, Toranchet A (1997) Risk factors of early menopause in two generations of gainfully employed French women. Maturitas 26(3): 165-74.

Chapuy MC, Arlot ME, Duboeuf F, Brun J, Crouzet B, Arnaud S, Delmas PD, Meunier PJ (1992) Vitamin D3 and calcium to prevent hip fractures in elderly women. New England Journal of Medicine 327: 1637-42.

Chatterjee R, Goldstone AH (1996) Gonadal damage and effects on fertility in adult patients with haematological malignancy undergoing stem cell transplantation. Bone Marrow Transplantation 17: 5-11.

Cheang A, Sitruk-Ware R, Samsioe G (1994) Transdermal oestradiol and cardiovascualr risk factors. British Journal of Obstetrics and Gynaecology 101: 571-81.

Chen FP, Chang SY (1997) Spontaneous pregnancy in patients with premature ovarian failure. Acta Obstetrica et Gynecologica Scandinavica 76(1): 81-2.

Chenoy R, Hussain S, Tayob Y, O'Brien PMS, Moss MY, Morse PF (1994) Effect of oral gamolenic acid from evening primrose oil on menopausal flushing. British Medical Journal 308: 501-3.

Chetkowski RJ, Meldrum DR, Steingold KA, Randle D, Lu JK, Eggena P, Hersham JM, Alkjaersig NK, Fletcher AP, Judd HL (1986) Biological effects of transdermal estradiol. New England Journal of Medicine 314(25): 1615-20.

Clark ST, Radford JA, Crowther D, Swindell R, Shalet SM (1995) Gonadal function following chemotherapy for Hodgkin's disease: a comparative study of MVPP and a seven-drug hybrid regimen. Journal of Clinical Oncology 13: 134-9.

Clunie G (1994) Osteoporosis prevention. British Journal of Hospital Medicine 52: 79-85.

Colditz GA, Hankinson SE, Hunter DJ, Willett WC, Manson JE, Stampfer MJ, Hennekens C, Rosner B, Speizer FE (1995) The use of estrogens and progestins and the risk of breast cancer in postmenopausal women. New England Journal of Medicine 332(24): 1589-93.

Collaborative Group on Hormonal Factors in Breast Cancer (1997) Breast cancer and hormone replacement therapy: collaborative reanalysis of data from 51 epidemiological studies of 52,705 women with breast cancer and 108,411 women without breast cancer. Lancet 350: 1047-59

Collins P (1996) Vascular aspects of estrogen. Maturitas 23: 217-26.

Cone FK (1993) Making Sense of Menopause. Fireside: Simon and Schuster.

Conway GS (1997) Premature ovarian failure. Current Opinions in Obstetrics and Gynecology 9: 202-6.

Conway GS, Hettiarachchi S, Murray A, Jacobs PA (1995) Fragile X permutations in familial premature ovarian failure. Lancet 346: 309-10.

Conway GS, Katlsas G, Patel A, Davies MC, Jacobs JS (1996) Characterization of idiopathic premature ovarian failure. Fertility and Sterility 65: 337-41.

Conway GS, Payne NN, Wegg J, Murray A, Jacobs PA (1998) Fragile X permutation-screening in women with premature ovarian failure. Human Reproduction 13: 1184-7.

Cook R, Golombok S, Bish A, Murray C (1995) Disclosure of donor insemination: parental attitudes. American Journal of Orthopsychiatry 65(4): 549-59.

Coope J, Coope J (1996) HRT, a general practice approach: How to reach the most vulnerable. British Journal of General Practice 50(1): 38-43.

Coope J, Marsh J (1992) Can we improve compliance with long-term HRT? Maturitas 15: 151-8.

Coope J, Roberts D (1990) A clinic for the prevention of osteoporosis in general practice. British Journal of General Practice 40: 295-9.

Coope J, Thomsom JM, Poller L (1975) Effects of 'natural oestrogen' replacement therapy on menopausal symptoms and blood clotting. British Medical Journal 4: 139-43.

Cooper A, Spencer C, Whitehead MI, Ross D, Barnard GJR, Collins WP (1998) Systemic absorption of progesterone from Progest cream in postmenopausal women. Lancet 351: 1255-6

Cooper-Hilbert B (1998) Infertility and Involuntary Childlessness: helping couples cope. New York: WW Norton.

Corenblum B, Rowe T, Taylor PJ (1993) High-dose, short-term glucocrticoids for the treatment of infertility resulting from premature ovarian failure. Fertility and Sterility 59: 988-91.

Cotton K (1992) Second Time Around: the full story of my second surrogate pregnancy. New Barnet: Kim Cotton,.

Coulam CB, Stringfellow S, Hoefnagel D (1983) Evidence for a genetic factor in the aetiology of premature ovarian failure. Fertility and Sterility 40: 693-5.

Cowan G, Warren LW, Young JL (1985) Medical perceptions of menopausal symptoms. Psychology of Women Quarterly 9: 3-13.

Craft I, Johnson MH, Sauer MV (1997) Education and debate. British Medical Journal 314: 1400-3.

Cramer DW; Huijuan Xu MPH, Harlow BL (1995) Family history as a predictor of early menopause. Fertility and Sterility 64(4): 740-5.

Critchley HO, Wallace WH, Shalet SM, Mamtora H, Higginson J, Anderson DC (1992) Abdominal irradiation in childhood: the potential for pregnancy. British Journal of Obstetrics and Gynaecology 99: 392-4.

Crockin SL (1997) Legally speaking. American Society for Reproductive Medicine News 31: 15-16.

Crosignani PG, Alagna F, Bolis PF, Dalpra L, Marozzi A, Nicolosi AE, Taborelli M, Terreni MG, Testa G, Tibiletti MG, Vegetti W (1998) Familial form of idiopathic premature and early menopause. Presented at the International Symposium of Ovarian Ageing, Brussels, Belgium. Abstract in International Journal of Fertility and Women's Medicine 43(4): 200.

Cummings SR, Eckert S, Krueger KA, Powles TJ, Cauley JA, Norton L, Nickelsen T, Bjarnaason NH, Morrow M, Lippman ME, Black D, Glusman JE, Costa A, Jordan VC (1999) [June 16] The effects of Raloxifene on risk of breast cancer in post menopausal women: results of the MORE randomised trial. JAMA 291(23): 2189-2197.

Daily Mail Sept 23 1999 'Surgeons Transplant Ovary to Reverse Menopause by Claudia Joseph and Kate Hurry p 1-2.

Daly E, Vessey MP, Hawkins MM, Carson JL, Gough P, Marsh S (1996) Risk of venous thromboembolism in users of hormone replacement therapy. Lancet 348: 977-80.

Daly J (1995) Caught in the web: the social construction of menopause as disease. Journal of Reproductive and Infant Psychology 13: 115-26.

Daniels K (1994) Adoption and donor insemination: factors influencing couples' choices. Child Welfare LXXIII 1: 5-14.

Daniels K (1997) Information sharing in gamete donation. In Let the Offspring Speak: discussion on donor conception. Donor Conception Support Group of Australia.

Daniluk JC (1988) Infertility: intrapersonal and interpersonal impact. Fertility and Sterility 49: 982-90.

Davies MC, Anderson MC, Mason B et al. (1990) Oocoyte donation: the role of endometrial receptivity. Human Reproduction 5: 862-9.

Davies MC, Hall ML, Jacobs HS (1990) Bone mineral loss in young women with amenorrhoea. British Medical Journal 301: 790-3.

Davis versus Davis (1989) WI. 140495.

Davis CJ, Davison RM, Conway GS (1998) Genetic basis of premature ovarian failure. Human Fertility 1: 20-2.

Davis DL (1986) The meaning of menopause in a Newfoundland fishing village. Culture, Medicine and Society 10: 73-94.

Davis SR (1996) Premature ovarian failure. Maturitas 23: 1-8.

Davison RM, Quilter CR, Webb J, Murray A, Fisher AM, Valentine A, Serhal P, Conway GS (1998) A familial case of X chromosome deletion ascertained by cytogenetic screening of women with premature ovarian failure. Human Reproduction 13: 3039-41.

Dawson-Hughes B, Dallal GE, Krall EA, Sadowski L, Sahyoun N, Tannenbaum S (1990) A controlled trial of the effect of calcium supplementation on bone density in postmenopausal women. New England Journal of Medicine 323: 878-83.

De Beauvoir S (1987) The Second Sex. Harmondsworth: Penguin.

Delmas PD, Bjarnason NH, Mitlak BH, Ravoux A, Shah AS, Huster WJ, Draper M, Christiansen C (1997) Effects of raloxifene on bone mineral density, serum cholesterol concentrations, and uterine endometrium in postmenopausal women. New England Journal of Medicine 337(23): 1641-7.

Denton E (1995) Breast cancer family history clinics: the Leicester experience. Journal of the British Menopause Society 1(2): 22-3.

Department of Health (1994) Nutritional aspects of cardiovascular disease. Report of the Cardiovascular Review Group committee on medical aspects of food policy. London: HMSO.

Department of Health (1998) Clinical examination of the breast. Circular issued to GPs.

Deutsch H (1925) In Roazen P (ed) Psychoanalysis of the Sexual Functions of Women. London: Karnac 1991. Originally: The menopause. International Journal of Psychoanalysis 65: 56-62 (1924).

Deutsch H (1945) The climacterium. In The Psychology of Women: a psychoanalytic interpretation, vol II. New York: Grune & Stratton, pp 456-91.

Deveraux LL, Hammerman AJ (eds) (1998) Infertility and Identity: new strategies for treatment. San Francisco, CA: Jossey Bass.

Dewhurst CJ, De Koos EB, Ferriera HP (1975) The resistant ovary syndrome. British Journal of Obstetrics and Gynaecology 82: 341-5.

Dickson GL (1990) A feminist poststructural analysis of the knowledge of menopause. Advances in Nursing Science 12: 15-31.

Diener E, Emmons RA, Larson RJ, Griffin S (1985) The Satisfaction with Life Scale. Journal of Personality Assessment 49: 71-6.

Domar AD, Broome A, Zuttermeister PC, Seibel M, Friedman R (1992) The prevalence and predictability of depression in infertile women. Fertility and Sterility 58(6): 1158-63.

Downey J, McKinney M (1992) The psychiatric status of women presenting for infertility evaluation. American Journal of Orthopsychiatry 62(2): 196-205.

Ebin V (1982) Interpretations of infertility, the Aowin people of south-west Ghana. In MacCormack CP (ed) Ethnography of Fertility and Birth. London: Academic Press.

Eden JA (1993) Menopause before 40 – premature but not always permanent. Australian and New Zealand Journal of Obstetrics and Gynaecology 33: 201-3.

Eichenbaum L, Orbach S (1983) Understanding Women. Harmondsworth: Penguin.

Erickson KT (1966) Wayward Puritans: a study of the sociology of deviance. New York: Wiley.

Erikson EH (1965) Childhood and Society. Harmondsworth: Penguin.

Ernst E (1999) Herbal remedies as a treatment of some frequent symptoms during the menopause. Journal of the British Menopause Society 5: 117-21.

Fallon AE, Rozin P (1985) Sex differences in perceptions of desirable body shape. Journal of Abnormal Psychology 94: 102-5.

Fallowfield L (1993) Giving sad and bad news. Lancet 34: 476-8.

Ferguson KJ, Hoegh C, Johnson S (1989) Estrogen replacement therapy: a survey of women's knowledge and attitudes. Archives of Internal Medicine 149: 133-6.

Finegold WJ (1976) Artificial Insemination with Husband's Sperm. Springfield, IL: Thomas, p 6.

Flint M (1975) The menopause: reward or punishment. Psychosomatics 16: 161-3.

Forna A (1998) Mother of all Myths: how society moulds and constrains mothers. London: Harper Collins.

Forrest L, Gilbert MS (1992) Infertility: an unanticipated and prolonged life crisis. Journal of Mental Health Counselling 14(1): 42-58.

Fox H (1992) The pathology of premature ovarian failure. Journal of Pathology 167: 357-63.

Francis RM, Anderson FH, Torgerson DJ (1995) A comparison of the effectiveness and cost of treatment for vertebral fractures in women. British Journal of Rheumatology 34: 1167-71.

Fraser IS, Shearman RP, Smith A, Russell P (1988) An association between blepharophimosis, resistant ovary syndrome and true menopause. Fertility and Sterility 50: 747-51.

Freeling P, Gask L (1998) Sticks and stones: changing terminology is no substitute for good consultation skills. British Medical Journal 317: 1028-9.

Freud S (1924) The Dissolution of the Oedipus Complex. In Penguin Freud Library, vol 7, pp 313-22. Harmondsworth: Penguin (1991).

Freud S (1937) Analysis terminable and interminable. Standard Edition 23. London: Hogarth Press (1955).

Gadducci A, Fanucchi A, Corsio S, Genazzani AR (1997) Hormone replacement therapy and gynecological cancer. Anticancer Research 17(5B): 3793-8.

Gangar K, Cust M, Whithead MI (1989) Symptoms of oestrogen deficiency associated with supraphysiological plasma oestradiol concentrations in women with oestradiol implants. British Medical Journal 299: 601-2.

Gannon L (1994) Sexuality and the menopause. In Choi PLY, Nicholson P (eds) Female Sexuality. London: Harvester Wheatsheaf.

Gannon L, Ekstrom B (1993) Attitudes toward menopause: the influence of sociocultural paradigms. Psychology of Women Quarterly 17(3): 275-88.

Gapstur SM, Morrow M, Sellers TA (1999) [June 9] Hormone Replacement Therapy and risk of breast cancer with a favourable histology: results of the IOWA Women's

Health Study. JAMA 281(22): 2091-2097.

Gilbert P (1992) Counselling for Depression. London: Sage.

Gilligan C (1982) In a Different Voice: psychological theory and women's development. Cambridge, MA: Harvard University Press.

Ginsburg J (1991) What determines the age at the menopause? British Medical Journal 302: 1288-9.

Ginsburg J, Prelevic GM (1995) Tibolone in postmenopausal women with a history of breast carcinoma. Journal of the British Menopause Society 1(2): 24-5.

Ginsburg J, Prelevic G, Butler D, Okolo S (1995) Clinical experience with tibolone (Livial) over 8 years. Maturitas 21: 71-7.

Goffman E (1959) The Presentation of Self in Everyday Life. Harmondsworth: Penguin.

Goldenberg H (1997) Who am I, if I am not a mother? In du Plock S (ed) Case Studies in Existential Psychotherapy and Counselling. Chichester: John Wiley.

Gosden R (1996) Cheating Time: science, sex and ageing. London: Macmillan.

Gosden RG, Baird DT, Wade JC, Webb R (1994) Restoration of fertility to oophorectomized sheep by ovarian autografts stored at -196 degree C. Human Reproduction 9:597-603.

Gosden RG, Faddy MJ (1998) Biological bases of premature ovarian failure. Reproduction Fertility Development 10(1): 73-8.

Gosden RG, Picton HM, Nugent D, Rutherford AJ (1999) 'Gonadal tissue cryopreservation: clinical objectives and practical prospects. Human Fertility 2: 107-114.

Gossain VV, Carella MJ, Rovner DR (1993) Case report: pregnancy in a patient with premature ovarian failure. Journal of Medicine 24(6): 393-02.

Greene JG (1983) Bereavement and social support at the climacteric. Maturitas 5: 115-25.

Greer G (1991) The Change. London: Hamish Hamilton.

Grodstein F, Stampfer MJ, Coldhaber SZ, Mansen JE, Colditz GA, Speizer FE, Willett WC, Hennekens CH (1996) Prospective study of exogenous hormones and risk of pulmonary embolism in women. Lancet 348: 983-7.

Grol R, de Maeseneer J, Whitfield M, Mokkink H (1990) Disease-centred versus patient-centred attitudes: comparison of general practitioners in Belgium, Britain and the Netherlands. Family Practice 7: 100-4.

Gulette MM (1997) Menopause as magic marker: discursive consolidation in the US and strategies for cultural combat. In Komesaroff P, Rothfield P, Daly J (eds) Reinterpreting Menopause: cultural and philosophical issues, pp 176-99. New York: Routledge.

Gutthann SP, Rodriguez LAG, Casjeusague J (1997) Hormone replacement therapy and risk of venous thromboembolism: population based case-control study. British Medical Journal 314: 796-800.

Hall J, Jacobs R (1991) Menopause Matters. Dorset: Element Books.

Hamblen EC (1939) Endocrine Gynaecology. Springfield, IL: Charles C Thomas, p 80.

Hammar M, Christau S, Nathorst-Boos J, Rud T, Garre K (1998) A double-blind randomised trial comparing the effects of tibolone and continuous combined hormone replacement therapy in postmenopausal women with menopausal symptoms. British Journal of Obstetrics and Gynaecology 105: 904-11.

Hampson SE, Hibbard JH (1996) Cross-talk about menopause: enhancing interactions about menopause and hormone therapy. Patient Education and Counselling 27: 177-84.

Harper J (1993) What does she look like? What children want to know about their birth parents. Adoption and Fostering 17(2): 27-9.

Harrar G, Sommer H (1994) Treatment of mild/moderate depression with hypericum. Phytomedicine 1: 3-8.

Harrison RF (1990) Stress in infertility. In Bonnar J (ed) Recent Advances in Obstetrics and Gynaecology. New York: Churchill Livingstone.

Hawkridge C (1997) My 20-year sticky patch. The Independent 13 May.

Hawton K, Salkovskis P, Kirk J, Clark DM (1989) Cognitive Behaviour Therapy for Psychiatric Problems. Oxford: Oxford University Press.

Headley JA, Theriault RL, LeBlanc AD, Vassilopoulou-Sellin R, Hortobagyi GN (1998) Pilot study of bone mineral density in breast cancer patients treated with adjuvant chemotherapy. Cancer Investigations 16(1): 6-11.

Health Alert: premature menopause (1997) Broadcasting Support Services.

Heinonen A, Kannus P, Sievanen H, Oja P, Pasanen M, Rinnen M, Uusi-Rasi K, Vuori I (1996) Randomised controlled trial of the effect of high impact exercise on selected risk factors for osteoporosis. Lancet 348: 1343-7.

Hendricks MC (1985) Feminist therapy with women and couples who are infertile. In Rosewater LB, Walker LEA (eds) Handbook of Feminist Therapy: women's issues in psychotherapy. New York: Springer.

Hendrix S (1997) Nonestrogen management of menopausal symptoms. Endocrinology and Metabolism Clinics of North America 26(2): 379-90.

HFEA and BMA (1996) Considering Surrogacy: your questions answered. London: HFEA and BMA.

Hibbard JH, Hampson SE (1993) Enhancing women's partnership with health providers in hormone replacement therapy decision-making: research and future directions. Journal of Women and Aging 52: 17-29.

Hickman TN, Namnoum AB, Hinton EL, Zacur HA, Rock JA (1998) Timing of estrogen replacement therapy following hysterectomy with oophorectomy for endometriosis. Obstetrics and Gynecology 91: 673-7.

Hillard T (1998) Quality of life after premature ovarian failure. Paper delivered at International Symposium of Ovarian Ageing. Brussels, Belgium. Abstract in International Journal of Fertility and Women's Medicine 43(4): 204-5.

Hoek A, Schoemaker J, Drexhage HA (1997) Premature ovarian failure and ovarian immunity. Endocrine Reviews 18(1): 107-34.

Holbrook SM (1990) Adoption, infertility and the new reproductive technologies: problems and prospects for social work and welfare policy. Social Work 35: 333-7.

Holte A (1992) Influences of natural menopause on health complaints; a prospective study of healthy Norwegian women. Maturitas 14(2): 127-41.

Hope S, Rees MCP (1995) Why do British women start and stop hormone replacement therapy? Journal of the British Menopause Society 1(2): 26-7.

Hope S, Wager E, Rees M (1998) Survey of British women's views on the menopause and HRT. Journal of the British Menopause Society 4(1): 33-6.

Horowitz MJ (1986) Stress Response Syndromes. Northvale, NJ: Aronson.

Hosking D, Chilvers CED, Christiansen C, Ravn P, Wasnich R, Ross P, McClung M, Balske A, Thompson D, Daley M, Yates AJ (1998) Prevention of bone loss with alendronate in postmenopausal women under 60 years of age. New England Journal of Medicine 338(8): 485-92.

Houghton D, Houghton P (1984) Coping with Childlessness. Guernsey: Unwin Hyman.

Howe D (1998) Patterns of Adoption. Oxford: Blackwell Science.

Hsueh AJ, Gellig H, Tsafriri A (1994) Ovarian follicle atresia: hormonally controlled apoptotic process. Endocrine Reviews 15: 707-24.

Huerta R, Mena A, Malacara J-M, Diaz-de-Leon J (1995) The symptoms at the menopausal and premenopausal years: their relationship with insulin, glucose, cortisol, FSH, prolactin, obesity and attitudes towards sexuality. Psychoneuroendocrinology 20(8): 851-64.

Hulley S, Grady D, Bush T, Furberg C, Hewrrington D, Riggs B, Vittinghoff E (1998) Randomized trial of estrogen plus progestin for secondary prevention of coronary heart disease in postmenopausal women. Journal of the American Medical Association 280: 605-13.

Hunt J, Monach JH (1997) Beyond the bereavement model: the significance of depression for infertility counselling. Human Reproduction 12(11) suppl. Journal of the British Fertility Society 2(2):188-94.

Hunter MS (1990) Emotional well-being, sexual behaviour and hormone replacement therapy. Maturitas 12: 299-314.

Hunter MS (1992) The South East England longitudinal study of the climacteric and postmenopause. Maturitas 14(2): 117-26.

Hunter MS (1994) Counselling in Obstetrics and Gynaecology. Leicester: BPS Books.

Hunter MS (1996) Editorial: Depression and the menopause. British Medical Journal 313: 1217-8.

Hunter MS, Liao KLM (1995) Problem solving groups for mid-aged women in general practice: a pilot study. Journal of Reproductive and Infant Psychology 13(2): 147-51.

Hunter MS, Liao KLM (1996) Evaluation of a four-session cognitive-behavioural intervention for menopausal hot flushes. British Journal of Health Psychology 1: 113-25.

Hunter MS, O'Dea I (1997) Menopause: bodily changes and multiple meanings. In Ussher JM (ed) Body Talk: the material and discursive regulation of sexuality, madness and reproduction. London: Routledge.

Hunter MS, O'Dea I (1999) Cognitive appraisal of the menopause: the development of the Menopause Representations Questionnaire (MRQ). (submitted).

Hunter MS, O'Dea I, Britten N (1997) Decision-making and hormone replacement therapy: a qualitative analysis. Social Science and Medicine 45: 1541-8.

Hutchon DJR , Cooper S (1998) Terminology for early pregnancy loss must be changed. British Medical Journal 317:1081.

Ireland M (1993) Reconceiving Women. New York: Guilford.

Israel D, Youngkin EQ (1997) Herbal therapies for perimenopausal and menopausal complaints. Pharmacotherapy 17(5): 970-84.

Jacobs PA (1991) Fragile X syndrome. Journal of Medical Genetics 28: 809-10.

Jacobson A, Galen DI, Weckstein LN (1991) Reproductive roulette: prognosis for ovarian failure. Fertility and Sterility 55(2): 446-7.

Jaeger AS (1996) Laws surrounding reproductive technologies. In Seibel MM, Crockin SI (eds) Family Building Through Egg and Sperm Donation. Sudbury, MA: Jones & Bartlett.

Jamin C, Sera B, Colau JC (1995) Pregnancy after the diagnosis of menopause. Contraception Fertilité Sexualité 23(11): 677-81.

Jensen J, Christiansen C, Rodbro P (1985) Cigarette smoking, serum estrogens, and bone loss during hormone replacement therapy early after menopause. New England Journal of Medicine 313(16): 973-5.

Jick H, Derby LE, Myers MW, Vasilakis C, Newton KM (1996) Risk of hospital admission for idiopathic venous thromboembolism among users of postmenopausal oestrogen. Lancet 348: 981-3.

Johnson CL (1996) Regaining self-esteem: strategies and interventions for the infertile woman. Journal of Obstetrics, Gynecologic and Neonatal Nursing 25:291-5.

Jones GS, Moraes-Rheusen M (1969) A new syndrome of amenorrhoea in association with hypergonadotropism and apparently normal ovarian follicular apparatus. American Journal of Obstetrics and Gynecology 104: 597-600.

Jones GS, Reuhsen M (1967) A new syndrome of amenorrhoea in association with hypogonadotropism and apparently normal follicular apparatus. Fertility and Sterility 18: 440.

Journal of British Menopause Society (1997) GP protocols for monitoring HRT in general practice. Journal of the British Menopause Society 3(4): 6.

Kanis JA, Powles T, Paterson AHG, McCloskey EV, Ashley A (1996) Clodrinate decreases the frequency of skeletal metastases in women with breast cancer. Bone 19 (6): 663-7.

Kaufert PA (1982) Myth and menopause. Society, Health and Illness 11: 141-66.

Kaufert PA, Gilbert P (1988) Researching the symptoms of the menopause; an exercise in methodology. Maturitas 10(2): 117-31.

Kaufert PA, Gilbert P, Tate R (1992) The Manitoba Project; a re-examination of the relationship between menopause and depression. Maturitas 14(2): 143-56.

Kaufert PA, Lock M (1997) Medicalisation of women's third age. Journal of Psychosomatic Obstetrics and Gynaecology 18(2): 81-7.

Kaufman FR, Reichardt JK, Ng WG, Xu YK, Manis FR, McBride Chang C, Wolff JA (1994) Correlation of cognitive, neurologic, and ovarian outcome with the Q188R mutation of the galactose-1-phosphate uridyltransferase gene. Journal of Pediatrics 125: 225-7.

Kenneson A, Cramer DW, Warren ST (1997) Fragile X permutations are not a major cause of early menopause. American Journal of Human Genetics 61(6): 1362-9.

Khamsi F, Endman MW, Lacanna IC, Wong J (1997) Some psychological aspects of oocyte donation from known donors on altruistic basis. Fertility and Sterility 68: 323-7.

Khaw K-T (1998) Hormone replacement Tterapy again: risk benefit relation differs between populations and individuals. British Medical Journal 316: 1842-4.

Killilea M (1976) Mutual help organisations: interpretations in the literature. In Caplan G, Killilea M (eds) Support Systems and Mutual Help: multi-disciplinary explorations. New York: Grune and Stratton.

Kirk HD (1984) Shared Fate: a theory and method of adoptive relationships, 2nd edn. Port Angeles, WA: Ben-Simon Publications.

Kirkland A, Power M, Burton G, Baber R, Studd J, Abdalla H (1992) Comparison of attitudes of donors and recipients to oocyte donation. Human Reproduction 7: 355-7.

Klein M (1946) Notes on some schizoid mechanisms. In Envy and Gratitude and Other Writings 1946-1963. London: Hogarth Press (1984).

Kloosterboer HJ, Deckers GH (1997) Tibolone and its metabolites: pharmacology, tissue specificity and effects in animal models of tumours. Gynaecology and Endocrinology 11(Suppl 1): 63-8.

Knight DC, Eden JA (1995) Phytoestrogens – a short review. Maturitas 22: 167-75.

Koch L (1998) Two decades of IVF: a critical appraisal. In Hildt E, Mieth D (eds) In vitro Fertilisation in the 1990s: towards a medical, social and ethical evaluation. Aldershot: Ashgate.

Komesaroff P, Rothfield P, Daly J (1997) Reinterpreting Menopause: cultural and philosophical issues. London: Routledge.

Komesaroff PA (1997) Medicine and the moral space of the menopausal woman. In Komesaroff P, Rothfield P, Daly J (eds) Reinterpreting Menopause. New York: Routledge.

Krafft-Ebbing R van (1877) Uber Imesin in Klimakterium. Psychiatry 34: 407.

Krall EA, Dawson-Hughes B (1991) Smoking and bone loss among postmenopausal women. Journal of Bone and Mineral Research 6: 331.

Kubler-Ross E (1970) On Death and Dying. London: Tavistock.

Ladipo P (1987) Women in a maize storage co-operative in Nigeria: family planning, credit and technological change. In Oppong C (ed) Sex Roles, Population and Development in West Africa: policy-related studies on work and demographic issues. Portsmouth, New Hampshire: Heinemann.

Laudenslager ML, Boccia ML, Reite ML (1993) Biobehavioral consequences of loss in nonhuman primates: Individual differences. In Stroebe MS, Stroebe W, Hansson RO (eds) Handbook of Bereavement: Theory, Research and Intervention, pp 129-42. Cambridge: Cambridge University Press.

Lauren (1998) Issues for donor-inseminated offspring. In Blyth E, Crawshaw M, Speirs J (eds) Truth and the Child 10 Years On: information exchange in donor assisted conception. Birminham: British Association of Social Workers Publications.

Lax RF (1982) The expectable depressive climacteric reaction. Bulletin of the Meninger Clinic 46: 151-67.

Lax RF (1997) The menopause phase: crisis, danger, opportunity. In On Becoming and Being a Woman. New York: Jason Aronson, pp 185-210.

Laya MB, Larson EB, Taplin SH, White E (1996) Effects of oestrogen replacement therapy on the specificity and sensitivity of screening mammography . Journal of the National Cancer Institute 88: 643-9.

Leadbetter A (1997) Hope in the freezer? (Readers' views) Progress in Reproduction 1(4): 2.

Lee JR (1990) Osteoporosis reversal. The role of progesterone. International Clinical Nutrition Review 10(3): 384-91.

Leiblum S (ed) (1997) Infertility: psychological issues and counselling strategies. Chichester: John Wiley.

Leick N, Davidsen-Nielsen M (1991) Healing Pain: attachment, loss and grief therapy. London: Routledge.

Lennon MC (1982) The psychological consequences of menopause: The importance of timing of a life stage event. Journal of Health and Social Behaviour 23: 353-66.

Lessor R, Reitz K, Balmaceda J, Asch RA (1991) Survey of public attitudes toward oocyte donation between sisters. Human Reproduction 5: 889-92.

Letterie GS, Bork MD, Miqazawa K (1990) Intermittent ovarian failure. Journal of Reproductive Medicine 35: 731-3.

Leventhal H, Nerenz D, Steele D (1984) Illness representations and coping with health threats. In Baum A, Singer J (eds) A Handbook of Psychology and Health, vol 4. New Jersey: Lawrence Earlbaum Associates.

Ley P (1982) Satisfaction, compliance and communication. British Journal of Clinical Psychology 21: 241-4.

Ley P (1988) Communicating with Patients. London: Croom Helm.

Liao KLM, Hunter MS (1994) The Women's Midlife Project: an evaluation of psychological services for mid-aged women in general practice. Clinical Psychology Forum 65: 19-22.

Liao KLM, Hunter MS (1998) Psychological effects. In Fraser I, Whitehead M (eds)

Estrogens and Progestogens in Clinical Practice. London: Churchill Livingstone.

Liao KLM, Hunter MS, White, P (1994) Beliefs about menopause of general practitioners and mid-aged women. Family Practice 11: 408-12.

Liao KLM, Wood N, Conway GS (1999) Premature ovarian failure and psychological health: descriptive data from a clinic sample. 2nd International Women and Health Conference. Edinburgh. (British Psychological Society Conference Abstracts).

Lieberman D, Kopernick G, Porath A, Laser S, Heimer D (1995) Sub-clinical worsening of bronchial asthma during estrogen replacement therapy in asthmatic postmenopausal women. Maturitas 21: 153-7.

Lindsey R, Hart D, McLean A, Clark A, Kraszewski A, Garwiid J (1978) Bone responcse to termination of estrogen treatment. Lancet 1: 1325-7.

Lock M (1991) Contested meanings of the menopause. Lancet 337: 1270-2.

Lock M, Kauffer P, Gilbert P (1988) Cultural construction of the menopausal symptom: the Japanese case. Maturitas 10: 317-22.

Luisetto G, Zangari M, Bottega F, Peccolo F, Galuppo P, Nardi A, Ziliotto D (1995) Different rates of forearm bone loss in healthy women with early or late menopause. Osteoporosis International 5(1): 54-62.

Luoh SW, Bain PA, Polankiewicz RD, Goodheart ML, Gardner H, Jaenisch R, Page DC (1997) ZFX mutations results in small animal size and reduced germ cell number in male and female mice. Development 124: 2275-84.

Luthra M (1997) Britain's Black Population: social change, public policy and agenda. Bodmin: Arena.

Lutjen P, Trounson A, Leeton J, Findlay J, Wood C, Renous P (1984) The establishment and maintenance of pregnancy using in vitro fertilisation and embryo donation in a patient with primary ovarian failure. Nature 307: 104-5.

McAllister F, Clarke L (1998) Choosing Childlessness. Family Policy Studies Unit Joseph Rowntree Foundation.

McCarthy T (1990) Menopause symptoms in Far Eastern countries – the Singapore segment. International Menopause Congress Abstract no. 018.

McCrea FB (1983) The politics of menopause: the discovery of a deficiency disease. Social Problems 31(1):1111-32.

McDermott EM, Powell RJ (1996) Incidence of ovarian failure in systemic lupus erythematosus after treatment with pulse cyclophosphamide. Annals of Rheumatic Diseases 55(4): 224-9.

McDonald M (1997) The cost of secrecy. In Let the Offspring Speak: discussion on donor conception. The Donor Conception Support Group of Australia.

McKinlay SM, Brambilla DJ, Posner JG (1992a) The normal menopause transition. Maturitas 14: 103-15.

McKinlay SM, Brambilla DJ, Posner JG (1992b) The normal menopausal transition. American Journal of Human Biology 4: 37-46.

McLaren HC (1949) Vitamin E in the menopause. British Medical Journal 2: 1378-80.

McLean S (1999) Old Law, New Medicine: Medical Ethics an Human Rights. London: Rivers Oram Press.

MacNaughton J, Banah M, McCloud P, Hee J, Burger HG (1992) Age related changes in follicle stimulating hormone, luteinizing hormone, oestradiol and immunoreactive inhibin in women of reproductive age. Clinical Endocrinology 36: 339-45.

MacPherson KI (1981) Menopause as a disease: the social construction of a metaphor. Advances in Nursing Science 3(2): 95-113.

McWhinnie AM (1996) Families following assisted conception: what do we tell our child? Department of Social Work, University of Dundee.

Maggs-Rapport F (1998) Miracles take a little longer. The Guardian (Society) 11 February: 2.

Maguire P (1985) Barriers to psychological care of the dying. British Medical Journal 291: 1711-13.

Mahadevan K, Murthy MSR, Reddy PR, Syamala Bhaskaran (1982) Early menopause and its determinants. Journal of Biosocial Science 14: 473-9.

Mahlstedt PP, Macduff S, Bernstein J (1987) Emotional factors and the in vitro fertilization and embryo transfer process. Journal of in Vitro Fertilization and Embryo Transfer 4: 232-6.

Manzi S, Meilahn EN, Rairie JE, Conte CG, Medsger TA Jr, Jansen-McWilliams L, D'Agostino RB, Keller LH (1997) Age-specific incidence rates of myocardial infarction and angina in women with systemic lupus erythematosus: comparison with the Framingham Study. American Journal of Epidemiology 145(5): 408-15.

Marsden J, Sacks NMP (1997) Tamoxifen and HRT: synergistic or antagonistic? Journal of the British Menopause Society 3(4): 9-17.

Marteau T (1994) Informed consent: methods of consent should be tested experimentally. British Medical Journal 308: 271-2.

Martin E (1987) The Woman in the Body. Milton Keynes: Open University Press.

Martin E (1990) Science and women's bodies: forms of anthropological knowledge. In Jacobus M, Keller EF, Shuttlework S (eds) Body/Politics: women and the discourses of science. London: Routledge.

Mashchak CA, Lobo RA, Dozono-Takano R, Eggana P, Brenner PF, Mishell Jr DR (1982) Comparison of pharmacodynamic properties of various estrogen formulations. American Journal of Obstetrics and Gynecology 144: 511-8.

Mashchak CA, Lobo RA, Dozono-Takano R, Eggana P, Brenner PF, Mishell Jr DR, Matthews KA, Schumaker SA, Bowen DJ, Langer RD, Hunt JR, Kaplan RM (1997) Women's Health Initiative: why now? What is it? What's new? American Psychologist 52: 101-16.

Matthews KA, Wing RR, Kuller LH (1990) Influences of natural menopause on psychological characteristics and symptoms of middle-aged healthy women. Journal of Consulting and Clinical Psychology 58: 345-63.

Mattison DR, Evans MI, Schwimmer MB, White BJ, Jensen B, Schulman JD (1984) Familial premature ovarian failure. American Journal of Human Genetics 36: 1341-48.

Medicines Control Agency (1996) Risk of venous thromboembolism with hormone replacement therapy. Committee on Safety of Medicines (CSM) 22: 9-10.

Mehta AE, Matwijiw I, Lyons EA, Faiman C (1992) Noninvasive diagnosis of resistant ovary syndrome by ultrasonography. Fertility and Sterility 57: 56-61.

Menage J (1994) Correspondence: Enforced hysterectomies. British Medical Journal 308:1574.

Merton RK, Fiske M, Kendall PJ (1990) The Focused Interview: a manual of problems and procedures, 2nd edn. New York: Free Press.

Miall CE (1987) The stigma of adoptive parent status: perceptions of community attitudes towards adoption and the experience of informal social sanctioning. Family Relations 36: 34-9.

Miller SM, Brody DS, Summerton J (1987) Styles of coping with threat: implications for health. Journal of Personality and Social Psychology 54: 142-8.

Mishell Jr DR (1982) Comparison of pharmacodynamic properties of various estrogen formulations. American Journal of Obstetrics and Gynecology 144: 511-8.

Mitchell J, Oakley A (1986) What is Feminism? Oxford: Blackwell.

Molly (1993) Letter. Registered Nurse 56(6): 11.

Money J, Ehrhart A (1972) Man and Woman, Boy and Girl. Baltimore, MD: Johns Hopkins University Press.

Moore DE, Kawagoe S, Davajan V, Nakamura RM, Mishell DR Jr (1978) An in vivo system in man for quantitation of estrogenicity. II. Pharmacologic changes in binding capacity of serum corticosteroid-binding globulin induced by conjugate estrogens, mestranol and ethynil estradiol. American Journal of Obstetrics and Gynecology 130: 475.

Moorey S, Greer S (1989) Psychological Therapy for Patients with Cancer: a new approach. Oxford: Heinemann Medical.

Moorhead T, Hannaford P, Warskyj M (1997) Prevalence and characteristics associated with use of hormone replacement therapy in Britain. British Journal of Obstetrics and Gynaecology 104: 290-7.

Morris SR, Sauer MV (1993) New advances in the treatment of infertility in women with ovarian failure. Current Opinion in Obstetrics and Gynecology 5: 368-77.

Mostyn B (1992) Infertility: Guidelines for Practice. London: Royal College of Obstetrics and Gynaecology Press.

Navot D, Drews MR, Bergh PA, Liusman I, Karstaedt A, Scott Jr RT, Garrisi GJ, Hofman GE (1994) Age related decline in female fertility is not due to diminished capacity of the uterus to sustain embryo implantation. Fertility and Sterility 61: 97-101.

Nelson LM, Anasti JN, Kimzey LM (1994) Development of luteinized graafian follicles in patients with karyotypically normal spontaneous premature ovarian failure. Journal of Clinical Endocrinology and Metabolism 79: 1470-5.

Neugarten B (1979) Time, age and the life cycle. American Journal of Psychiatry 136: 887-94.

Neugarten BL, Wood V, Kraines RJ, Loomis B (1968) Women's attitudes toward the menopause. In Neugarten BL (ed) Middle Age and Aging, pp 195-200. Chicago, IL: University of Chicago Press.

Neustatter A (1997) HRT or not HRT? The Guardian G2 14 October: p.]4.

Newton H, Aubard Y, Rutherford A, Sharma V, Gosden R (1996) Low temperature storage and grafting of human ovarian tissue. Human Reproduction 11: 1487-91.

Nielson L (1996) Procreative tourism, genetic testing and the law. In Lowe N, Douglas G (eds) Families Across Frontiers. The Hague: Martinus Nijhoff.

Notman N (1984) Psychiatric disorders at menopause. Psychiatric Annals 14: 448-53.

Notman N (1995) Reproductive and critical transitions in the lifespan of women patients with a focus on menopause. In Depression. Cambridge, MA: Harvard Medical School, pp 99-106.

O'Connor N, Ryan J (1993) Wild Desires and Mistaken Identities: lesbianism and psychoanalysis. London: Virago.

O'Donnell M (1991) Sociology in Focus: race and ethnicity. New York: Longman.

O'Herlihy C, Pepperell RJ, Evans JH (1980) The significance of FSH elevation in young women with disorders of ovulation. British Medical Journal 281: 1447-50.

Okon MA, Lee S, Li TC (1997) Period-free hormone replacement therapy. Journal of the British Menopause Society 3(1): 11-14.

Oktay K, Newton H, Aubard Y, Salha O, Gosden RG (1988) Cryopreservation of immature human oocytes and ovarian tissue: an emerging technology? Fertility and Sterility 69:1-7.

Oldenhave A (1991) Well-being and Sexuality in the Climacteric. Geneva: International Health Foundation.

Oleson T, Flocco W (1993) Randomised controlled study of premenstrual symptoms treated with ear, hand and foot reflexology. Obstetrics and Gynecology 82(6): 906-11.

Olivar AC (1996) The role of laparoscopic ovarian biopsy in the management of premature gonadal failure. Connecticut Medicine 60(12): 707-8.

Oppong C (1987) Sex Roles, Population and Development in West Africa: policy-related studies on work and demographic issues. Portsmouth, NH: Heinemann.

Orbach S (1998a) The cruel fact is that most women want to change something about their bodies: they are dissatisfied, hypercritical. The Guardian (Women's section) 10 February: p.4.

Orbach S (1998b) Hearts and minds: girls no longer feel down about busting up. The Guardian G2: p.7.

Orbach S, Eichenbaum L (1995) From objects to subjects. British Journal of Psychotherapy 12(1): 89-97.

Pados G, Camus M, Van Steirteghem A, Bonduelle M, Devroey P (1994) The evolution and outcome of pregnancies from oocyte donation. Human Reproduction 9: 538-42.

Palmlund I (1997) The marketing of estrogens for menopausal and postmenopausal women. Journal of Psychosomatic Obstetrics and Gynaecology 18(2): 158-64.

Panel report (1996) Psychoanalytic aspects of menopause, Spring APA 1994. Journal of the American Psychoanalytic Association 44: 631-8.

Panidis D, Rousso D, Vavilis D, Skiadopoulos S, Kalogeropoulos A (1994) Familial blepharophimosis with ovarian dysfunction. Human Reproduction 9: 2034-7.

Parker PJ (1984) Surrogate motherhood, psychiatric screening and informed consent, baby selling, and public policy. Bulletin of the American Academy of Psychiatry and the Law 12: 21.

Parkes CM (1972) Bereavement: studies of grief in adult life. Harmondsworth: Penguin.

Parlee M (1976) Social factors in the psychology of menstruation, birth and menopause. Primary Care 3: 477-90.

Parrot DM (1960) The fertility of mice with orthotopic grafts derived from frozen tissue. Journal of Reproduction and Fertility 1: 230-41.

Paulson RJ, Hatch IE, Lobo RA et al. (1997) Cumulative conception and live birth rates after oocyte donation: implicaitons regarding endometrial receptivity. Human Reproduction 12: 835-9.

Payer L (1991) The menopause in various cultures. In Burger H, Boulet M (eds) A Portrait of the Menopause. Carnforth, Lancs: Parthenon.

Pearce J, Hawton K, Blake F (1995) Psychological and sexual symptoms associated with the menopause and the effects of hormone replacement therapy: a review. British Journal of Psychiatry 167: 167-3.

Pennell Report on women's health (1998) The Pennell Initiative, Health Services Management Unit, University of Manchester: Laurence Chung Ltd.

PEPI Trial Writing Group (1996) Effects of hormone therapy on bone mineral density. Journal of the American Medical Association 276(17): 1389-96.

Perloff WA, Schneeberg NG (1957) The premature climacterium. American Practitioners' Digest of Treatments 8: 1955.

Person E, Ovesey L (1983) Psychoanalytic theories of gender identity. Journal of the American Academy of Psychoanalysis 11: 203-26.

Peterson AC, Crockett LJ (1985) Pubertal timing and grade effects on adjustment. Journal of Youth and Adolescence 14: 191-206.

Petrie K, Weinman J (1997) Perceptions of Health and Illness. Amsterdam: Harwood Academic Publishers.

Petrie P (1990) The Adolescent Years: a guide for parents. London: Michael Joseph.

Phoenix A, Woollett A, E Lloyd (eds) (1991) Motherhood, Meanings, Practices and Ideologies. London: Sage.

Pines D (1993) The menopause. In A Woman's Unconscious Use of Her Body: a psychoanalytical perspective. London: Virago, pp 151-66.

Pines M (1995) The universality of shame: a psychoanalytic approach. British Journal of Psychotherapy 11(13): 346-57.

Piringer P, Agana-Defensor R, Mullen N, Lee L (1993) A model for the development and implementation of a patient support group in a medical-surgical setting. Holistic Nursing Practice 8 (1): 16-25.

Poller L, Thomson JM, Coope J (1977) Conjugated equine estrogens and blood clotting: a follow-up report. British Medical Journal 1: 935-6.

Potter J, Wetherell M (1987) Discourse and Social Psychology: beyond attitudes and beliefs. London: Sage.

Powell CM, Taggart RT, Drumhjeller TC, Wangsa D, Qian C, Nelson LM , White BJ (1994) Molecular and cytogenetic studies of an X-autosome translocation in a patient with premature ovarian failure and review of the literature. American Journal of Medical Genetics 52: 19-26.

Power M, Baber R, Abdalla H, Kirkland A, Leonard T, Studd JWW (1990) A comparison of the attitudes of volunteer donors and infertile patient donors on an ovum donation programme. Human Reproduction 5: 352-5.

Powles TJ, Hickish T, Casey S, O'Brien M (1993) Hormone replacement after breast cancer. Lancet 342: 60.

Powles TJ, Jones AL, Ashley SE (1994) The Royal Marsden Hospital pilot tamoxifen chemoprevention trial. British Cancer Research and Treatment 31: 73-82.

Prince RL, Smith M, Dick IM, Price RI, Webb PG, Henderson NK, Harris MM (1991) Prevention of osteoporosis. A comparative study of exercise, calcium supplementation and hormone replacement therapy. New England Journal of Medicine 325: 1189-95.

Pyorala K, De Backer G, Graham I et al. (1994) Prevention of coronary heart disease in clinical practice. European Heart Journal 15:1300-31.

Rachman S (1980) Emotional processing. Behaviour Research and Therapy 18: 51-60.

Radford T (1998) How to live longer. The Guardian 16 January: p.17.

Radloff L (1977) The CES-D Scale: a self-report depression scale for research in the general population. Applied Psychosocial Measurement 1: 385-401.

Raphael-Leff (1995) Imaginative bodies of childbearing: visions and revisions. In Erskine A, Judd D (eds) The Imaginative Body – psychodynamic therapy in healthcare. London: Whurr.

Raphael-Leff (1997) The casket and the key: thoughts on gender and generativity. In Raphael-Leff J, Perelberg RJ (eds) Female Experience: three generations of British female psychoanalysts on their work with female patients, pp 237-57. London: Routledge.

Raudaskoski TH, Lahti EI, Kauppila AJ, Apaja-Sarkkinen MA, Laatikainen TJ (1995) Transdermal oestrogen with a levonorgestrel-releasing intrauterine device for climacteric complaints: clinical and endometrial responses. American Journal of Obstetrics and Gynecology 172(1): 114-19.

Ravn P, Lind C, Nilas L (1995) Lack of influence of simple premenopausal hysterectomy on bone mass and bone metabolism. American Journal of Obstetrics and Gynecology 172: 891-5.

Ravnikar VA (1987) Compliance with hormone therapy. American Journal of Obstetrics and Gynecology 156: 1332-4.

Rebar RW (1982) Hypergonadotrphic amenorrhoea and premature ovarian failure. Journal of Reproductive Medicine 27: 179-86.

Reitz R (1987) Menopause: a positive approach. Dallas, PA: Penguin.

Reitz R (1991) Foreword. In Taylor D, Sumrall AC (eds) Women of the 14th Moon, pp xi-xiv. Freedom, CA: Crossing Press.

Rice PL (1995) Pog Laus Tsis Khaub Hcaws Lawm: the Meaning of Menopause in Hmong Women. Journal of Reproductive and Infant Psychology 3: 79-92.

Rich C (1992) Ageing, ageism and feminist avoidance. In Crowley H, Himmelweit S (eds) Knowing Women. Milton Keynes: Open University Press.

Richters JMA (1997) Menopause in different cultures. Journal of Psychosomatic Obstetrics and Gynaecology 18(2): 73-80.

Roberts P-J (1995) Reported satisfaction among women receiving hormone replacement therapy in a dedicated general practice clinic and in a normal consultation. British Journal of General Practice 45: 79-81.

Robertson J (1989) Ethical and legal issues in human egg donation. Fertility and Sterility 52: 353-63.

Robinson D (1980) Self-help health groups. In Smith PB (ed) Small Groups and Interpersonal Change. London: Methuen.

Rosenberg M (1979) Conceiving the Self. New York: Basic Books.

Rosenwaks Z, Davis OK, Damario MA (1995) The role of maternal age in assisted reproduction. Human Reproduction 10: 165-73.

Roter D (1989) Which facets of communications have strong effects on outcome: a meta-analysis. In Stewart M, Roter D (eds) Communicating with Medical Patients. Newbury Park: Sage.

Rothert M (1991) Perspectives and issues in studying patient's decision-making. Proceedings of the AHCPR Conference on Primary Care Research: Theory and Methods. US Department of Health and Human Services, pp 175-9.

Rothert M, Padonu G, Holmes-Rovner M, Kroll J, Talarczyk G, Rovner D, Schmitt N, Breer L. (1994) Menopausal women as decision-makers in health care. Experimental Gerontology 29: 463-8.

Rothfield P (1997) Menopausal embodiment. In: Komesaroff P, Rothfield P, Daly J (eds) Reinterpreting Menopause. New York: Routledge.

Rowland R (1987) Technology and motherhood: reproductive choice reconsidered. Signs: Journal of Women in Culture and Society 12(3): 512-28.

Rubin SS (1993) The death of a child is forever: the life course impact of child loss. In Stroebe MS, Stroebe W, Hansson RO (eds) Handbook of Bereavement: theory, research and intervention, pp 285-99. Cambridge: Cambridge University Press.

Sadler AG, Syrop CH (1987) The stress of infertility: recommendations for assessment and intervention. Family Therapy Case Studies 22: 1-17.

Sala C, Arrigo G, Torri G, Martinazzi F, Riva P, Larizza L, Philippe C, Jonveaux P, Sloan F, Labella T, Toniolo D (1997) Eleven X chromosome breakpoints associated with premature ovarian failure (POF) map to a 15-Mb YAC contig spanning Xq21. Genomics 40: 123-31.

Salkovskis PM (ed) (1996) Frontiers of Cognitive Therapy. New York: Guildford Press.

Salzer LP (1991) Surviving infertility: a compassionate guide through the emotional crisis of infertility, revised edn. New York: Harper Collins.

Sanchez-Guerrero J, Liang MH, Karlson EW, Hunter DJ, Colditz GA (1995) Postmenopausal estrogen therapy and the risk for developing systemic lupus erythematosus. Annals of Internal Medicine 122(6): 430-3.

Sandelowski M (1991) Compelled to try: the never-enough quality of conceptive technology. Medical Anthropology Quarterly 5: 129-47.

Sandelowski M, Harris BG, Holditch-Davis D (1989) Mazing: infertile couples and the quest for a child. Image: Journal of Nursing Scholarship 21: 220-6.

Santen R, Pritchard K, Burger H (eds) 1998 Treatment of estrogen deficiency symptoms in women surviving breast cancer. Obstetrical and Gynecological Survey 53(10) Suppl: S1-S83.

Sauer MV (1996) Oocyte donation: reflection on past work and future directions. Human Reproduction 11: 1149-50.

Sauer MV, Paulson RJ, Lobo RA (1990) A preliminary report on oocyte donation extending reproductive potential to women over 40. New England Journal of Medicine 323: 1157.

Sauer MV, Paulson RJ, Lobo RA (1995) Pregnancy in women 50 or more years of age: outcomes of 22 consecutively established pregnancies from oocyte donation. Fertility and Sterility 64: 111-15.

Sauer MV, Paulson RJ, Moyer DL (1997) Assessing the importance of endometrial biopsy prior to oocyte donation. J Assis Reprod Genet 14: 125-7.

Sayers J (1988) Anorexia, Psychoanalysis and Feminism: fantasy and reality. Journal of Adolescence 11: 361-71.

Scambler A, Scambler G (1993) Menstrual Disorders. London: Tavistock/Routledge.

Schiffman R, Tedeschi G, Kinkel RP, Trapp BD, Frank JA, Kaneski CR, Brady RO, Barton NW, Nelson L, Yanovski JA (1997) Leukodystrophy in patients with ovarian dysgenesis. Annals of Neurology 41(5): 654-61.

Schneider-Gadicke A, Beer-Romero P, Brown LG Nussbaum R, Page DC (1989) ZFX has a gene structure similar to ZFY, the putative human sex determinant, and escapes X inactivation. Cell 57: 1247-58.

Schover LR (1994) Sexuality and body image in younger women with breast cancer. Monograph. National Cancer Institute 16: 177-82.

Schwartz LB, Chiu AS, Courtney M, Krey L, Schmidt-Sarosi C (1997) The embryo versus endometrium controversy revisited as it relates to predicting pregnancy outcome in in vitro fertilization-embry transfer cycles. Human Reproduction 12: 45-50.

Seeley T (1992) Oestrogen replacement therapy after hysterectomy. British Medical Journal 305: 811-12.

Sethi K, Pitkin J (1995) HRT uptake and compliance. European Journal of the Menopause 2(4): 33-4.

Sharpe S (1994) Just Like A Girl: how girls learn to be women: from the seventies to the nineties. Harmondsworth: Penguin.

Showalter E (1987) The Female Malady. London: Virago.

Siddle N, Sarrel P, Whitehead M (1987) The effect of hysterectomy on the age of ovarian failure. Fertility and Sterility 47: 94-100.

Silbergeld EK, Flaws JA (1999) Chemicals and menopause: effects on age at menopause and on health status in the postmenopausal period. Journal of Women's Health 8(2): 227-34.

Silver RC, Wortman CB (1991) Coping with undesirable life events. In Monat A, Lazarus R (eds) Stress and Coping: an anthology. New York: Columbia University Press.

Simons HF (1995) Wanting Another Child: coping with secondary infertility. San Francisco, CA: Jossey-Bass.

Singer D (1996) Premature menopause: the sense of self and social discourse. MA thesis, City University.

Singer D, Hunter M (1999) The experience of premature menopause: a thematic discourse analysis. Journal of Reproductive and Infant Psychology 17(1): 63-81.

Singh RP, Carr DH (1966) The anatomy and histology of XO human embryos and fetuses. Anatomical Record 155: 369-83.

Slade P, Emery J, Lieberman BA (1997) A prospective, longitudinal study of emotions and relationships in in-vitro fertilization treatment. Human Reproduction 12(1): 183-90.

Smith JA, Harre R, Van Langenhove L (1995) Idiography and the case study. In Smith JA, Harre R, Van Langenhove L (eds) Rethinking Psychology. London: Sage.

Smith RL (1956) Recorded and expected mortality among the Japanese of the United States and Hawaii, with special refernce to cancer. Journal of the National Cancer Institute 17: 459-73.

Soderstrom-Anttila V, Hovatta O (1995) An oocyte donation program with goserelin down-regulation of voluntary donors. Acta Obstetrica et Gynecologica Scandinavica 74: 288-92.

Spitzer WO (1997) The 1995 Pill scare revisited: anatomy of a non-epidemic. Human Reproduction 12(11): 2339-40, 2347-57.

Stampfer MK, Colditz GA, Willett WC, Manson JE, Rosner B, Speizer FE, Hennekens CH (1991) Post-menopausal estrogen therapy and cardiovascular disease: ten year follow-up from the Nurse's Health Study. New England Journal of Medicine 325: 756-62.

Starup J, Sele V (1973) Premature ovarian failure. Acta Obstetrica et Gynecologica Scandinavica 52: 259.

Steinem G (1981) Outrageous Acts and Everyday Rebellions. New York: Holt, Rinehart and Winston.

Stepanich KK (1992) Sister Moon Lodge: the power and mystery of menstruation. St Paul, MN: Llewellyn Publications.

Stolberg SG (1998) Quandary on donor eggs: what to tell the children. New York Times 18 January.

Stoller RJ (1985) Presentations of Gender. New Haven, CT: Yale University Press.

Stomper PC, Bradley J, Van Voorhis BJ, Ravnikar VA, Meyer JE (1990) Mammographic changes associated with postmenopausal hormone replacement therapy: a longitudinal study. Radiology 174: 487-90.

Suissa S, Blais L, Spitzer WO, Cusson J, Lewis M, Heinemann L (1997) First time use of newer oral contraceptives and the risk of venous thromboembolism. Contraception 56: 141-6.

Sullivan JM, Vander Zwang R, Hughes JP, Maddock V, Kroetz FW, Ramanathan KB, Mirvis DM (1990) Estrogen replacement and coronary artery disease:effect on survival in postmenopausal women. Archives of Internal Medicine 150(12): 2257-62.

Sung L, Bustillo M, Mukherjee T, Booth G, Karstaedt A, Copperman AB (1997) Sisters of women with premature ovarian failure may not be ideal ovum donors. Fertility and Sterility 67(5): 912-16.

Sybylla R (1997) Situating menopause within the strategies of power. In Komesaroff P, Rothfield P, Daly J (eds) Reinterpreting Menopause: cultural and philosophical issues. London: Routledge.

Tanna N (1999) Pharmacists and the management of the menopause. The Journal of the British Menopause Society. 5(2): 87.

Tanna NK, Pitkin J (1997) Monitoring patients on HRT within the primary care setting. Journal of the British Menopause Society 3(3): 11-15.

Taylor M (1997) Alternatives to conventional hormone replacement therapy. Complementary Therapy 23(8): 514-32.

Templeton A, Morris JK, Parslow W (1996) Factors that affect outcome of in-vitro fertilisation treatment. Lancet 348: 1402.

Tham DM, Gardner CD, Haskell WL (1998) Potential health benefits of dietary phytoestrogens: a review of the clinical, epidemiological, and mechanistic evidence. Journal of Clinical Endocrinology and Metabolism 83: 2223-5.

Tiggemann M, Pennington B (1990) The development of gender differences in body size dissatisfaction. Australian Psychologist 25: 306-13.

Tilt EJ (1870) The Change of Life in Health and Disease. London: John Churchill.

Tobin-Richards MH, Boxer AM, Peterson A (1983) The psychological significance of pubertal change: sex differences in perceptions of self during early adolescence. In Brooks-Gunn J, Peterson A (eds) Girls at Puberty: biological and psychosocial perspectives. New York: Plenum.

Toozs-Hobson P, Cardozo L (1996) Hormone replacement therapy for all? Universal prescription is desirable. British Medical Journal 313: 350-2.

Torgerson DJ, Thomas RE, Reid DM (1997) Mothers' and daughters' menopasual ages: is there a link? European Journal of Obstetrics, Gynecology and Reproductive Biology 74(1): 63-6.

Triseliotis J (1973) In Search of Origins. London: Routledge & Kegan Paul.

Trounson A, Leeton J, Besanko M, Wood C, Conti A (1983) Pregnancy established in an infertile patient after of a donated embryo fertilised in vitro. British Medical Journal 286: 835-8.

Trounson A, Mohr L (1983) Human pregnancy following cryopreservation, thawing and transfer of an eight cell embryo. Nature 305:707-9.

Tulandi T, Kinch RAH (1981) Premature Ovarian Failure. Obstetrical and Gynecological Survey Supplement 36(9): 521-527.

Tyson P, Tyson RL (1990) Psychoanalytic Theories of Development: an integration. New Haven: Yale University Press.

Ussher JM (1989) The Psychology of the Female Body. London: Routledge.

Ussher JM (1992) Reproductive rhetoric and the blaming of the body. In Nicolson P, Ussher J (eds) The Psychology of Women's Health and Health Care. London: Macmillan.

Ussher JM (1997a) Fantasies of Femininity: betraying the boundaries of sex. Harmondsworth: Penguin.

Ussher JM (1997b) Body Talk: the material and discursive regulation of sexuality, madness and reproduction. London: Routledge.

Van Balen F, Verdurmen J, Ketting E (1997) Choices and motivation of infertile couples. Patient Education and Counselling 31: 19-27.

Veevers J (1980) Childless by Choice. Toronto: Butterworths.

Veevers JE (1972) The violation of fertility mores: voluntary childlessness as deviant behaviour. In Boydell CCL, Grindstaff CF, Whitehead PC (eds) Deviant Behaviour and Societal Reaction, pp 571-92. Toronto: Holt, Rhinehart and Winston.

Vegetti W, Tibiletti M, Testa G, Yankowski L, Alagna F, Castoldi E, Taborelli M, Motta T, Bolis PF, Dalpra L, Crosignani PG (1998) Inheritance in idiopathic premature ovarian failure: analysis of 71 cases. Human Reproduction 13: 1796-800.

Vermeulen A (1993) Environment, human reproduction, menopause and andropause. Environmental Health Perspectives Supplements 101(suppl 2): 91-100.

Vinatier D, Dufour P, Tordjeman-Rizzi N, Prolongeau JF, Depret-Moser S, Monnier JC (1995) Immunological aspects of ovarian function: role of the cytokines. European Journal of Obstetrics, Gynecology and Reproductive Biology 63(2): 155-68.

Warnock M (1998) The Intelligent Person's Guide to Ethics. London: Duckworth.

Watson NR, Studd JWW (1993) Bone loss following hysterectomy with ovarian conservation. European Journal of Obstetrics, Gynecology and Reproductive Biology 49: 87.

Webb P (1997) British Homeopathic Association. The Family Encyclopedia of Homeopathic Remedies. London: Robinson Publishing, pp 488-94.

Weetman AP (1995) Autoimmunity to steroid-producing cells and familial polyendocrine autoimmunity. Baillières Clinical Endocrinology and Metabolism 9: 157-74.

Weiner B (1992) Human Motivation: metaphors, theories and research. Newbury Park, CA: Sage.

Welldon E (1988) Mother, Madonna, Whore: the idealisation and denigration of motherhood. London: Free Association.

Wheeler CA (1995) Premature ovarian failure: treatment strategies. Reproductive and Immunological Medicine 76(5): 130-1.

Whipp C (1998) The legacy of deceit: a donor offspring's perspective on secrecy in assisted conception. In Blyth E, Crawshaw M, Speirs J (eds) Truth and the Child 10 Years On: information exchange in donor assisted conception. Birmingham: British Association of Social Workers Publications.

Whiteford LM, Gonzles L (1994) Stigma: the hidden burden of infertility. Social Science Medicine 40(1): 27-36.

Wilbush J (1979) La menespausie – the birth of a syndrome. Maturitas 1: 145-57.

Willis DB, Calle EE, Miracle-McMahill HL, Heath CW (1996) Estrogen replacement therapy and risk of fatal breast cancer in a prospective cohort of postmenopausal women in the United States. Cancer Causes and Control 7: 449-57.

Wilson RA (1966) Feminine Forever. New York: Evans.

Winston R (1986) Infertility: a sympathetic approach. London: Optima 1995.

Witteman JCM, Grobbee DE, Kok FJ, Jofman A, Valkenburg HA (1989) Increased risk of atherosclerosis in women after the menopause. British Medical Journal 298: 642-4.

Wood C (1975) Mumps and the menopause. British Journal of Sexual Medicine 2: 19.

Wood CE, Shaw JM, Trounson AO (1997) Cryopreservation of ovarian tissue: potential 'reproductive insurance' for women at risk of early ovarian failure. Medical Journal of Australia 166(7): 366-9.

Wood N (1996) The Psychological Aspects of Premature Menopause: an exploratory study. MA thesis, University College London.

Woodfield RL, Viney LL (1982) Bereavement: a personal construct approach. Cited in Raphael B (1990) The Anatomy of Bereavement: a handbook for the caring professions. London: Routledge.

Woodham A (1994) HEA guide to Complementary medicine and therapy. London: Health Education Authority, pp 1-13.

Woolf V (1937) Quoted in AO Bell (ed) Diary of Virginia Woolf, vol 5, 1936-41. London: Chatto & Windus (1984).

Woollett A (1995) Questioning 'motherhood' as a model for women's lives and development. Paper presented at Women and Psychology Conference, University of Leeds.

Worcester N, Whatley MH (1992) The selling of HRT: playing the fear factor. Feminist Review 41: 1-26.

World Health Organization Group (1996) Research on the menopause in the 1990s. WHO Technical Report Series 866.

Wyon Y, Lindgren R, Lundeberg T, Hammar M (1995) Effects of acupuncture on climacteric vasomotor symptoms, quality of life, and urinary excretion of neuropeptides among postmenopausal women. Journal of the North American Menopause Society 2(1): 3-12.

Yalom I (1980) The Theory and Practice of Group Psychotherapy. New York: Basic Books.

Yorburg B (1974) Sexual Identity; sex roles and social change. New York: John Wiley.

Younis JS, Simon A, Laufer N (1996) Endometrial preparation: lessons from oocyte donation. Fertility and Sterility 66: 873-84.

Yovich J, Blackledge D, Richardson P, Matson P, Turner S, Draper R (1987) Pregnancies following pronuclear stage tubal transfer. Fertility and Sterility 48: 851.

Zachary A (1995) Narcissism in ageing. In Cooper J, Maxwell N (eds.) Narcissistic Wounds: clinical perspectives, pp 94-100. London: Whurr.

Zarate A, Karchmer S, Gomez E, Castelazo AL (1970) Premature menopause: a clinical, histological and cytogenetic study. American Journal of Obstetrics and Gynecology 106: 110.

Zinn AR, Page DC, Fisher EMC (March 1993) Turner syndrome: the case of the missing sex chromosome. Trends in Genetics 9: 90-3.

Resources

Leaflets

Breast Awareness
Women's Nationwide Cancer Control Campaign
128 Curtain Road
London EC2
Tel: 020 7729 4688

Health Alert: premature menopause
PO Box 4000
London W12 8UF
or Cardiff CF5 2XT

Support groups

Early Menopause Support Group
Janet Wainwright Wing
King's College Hospital
Denmark Hill
London SE5 9RS
Tel: 020 7346 3336

Northwick Park & St Mark's NHS Trust
c/o Dani Singer
Northwick Park Hospital
Watford Road
Harrow
Middlesex HA1 3UJ
Tel: 020 8869 2877
Fax: 020 8869 2009

Premature Menopause Support Group (formerly Daisychain)
PO Box 392
High Wycombe
Buckinghamshire HP15 7SH
http://www.daisychain.org. uk
Self-help group with membership newsletter and telephone linkline for support

Premature Menopause Support Group (NZ)
c/o Dr Andrew Shelling
Department of Obstetrics and Gynaecology
National Women's Hospital
Claude Road
Auckland

Organizations

Amarant Trust
80 Lambeth Road
London SE1 7PW
Tel: 020 7401 3855
Charity set to up to research the menopause and provide information and advice, particularly in relation to HRT. Provides advice on treatment, information and leaflets including one on premature menopause
Advice line run by a doctor and a team of nurses 11 am to 6 pm each weekday, tel: 01293 413000
Also has series of 24-hour helplines on 0891 660 620; information about alternatives to HRT on 0891 660 630; details of new (HRT) treatments on 0891 660631
Phone lines charged at premium rates

British Acupuncture Council
Park House
206-208 Latimer Road
London W10 6RE
Tel: 020 8964 0222
Fax: 020 8964 0333
e-mail: info@acupuncture.org.uk
Provides list of accredited pratitioners and general information leaflet

British Agency for Adoption and Fostering (BAAF)
Skyline House
200 Union Street
London SE1 0LX
Tel: 020 7593 2000 (HQ)
Tel: 020 7928 6085 (South Regional Centre)
Gives information and advice, and produces information leaflets and books

British Association of Counselling (BAC)
1 Regent Place
Rugby
Warwickshire CV21 2PJ
Tel: 01788 550899
Fax: 01788 562189
minicom: 01788 572838
e-mail: bac@bac.co.uk
Accredited members have experience of a wide range of counselling. Write enclosing a stamped self-addressed envelope for a list of counsellors in your area

British Association of Psychotherapists (BAP)
37 Mapesbury Road
London NW2 4HJ
Tel: 020 8452 9823
Fax: 020 8452 5182

British Fertility Society
c/o P Wardle
Honorary Secretary
Division of Obstetrics and Gynaecology
Department of Hospital Medicine
Level D
St Michael's Hospital
Bristol BS2 8EG
Tel: 0117 928 5624
Fax: 0117 927 2792
Newsletter web site: http://www.ReproMED.org.uk/BFS/

British Homeopathic Association
27a Devonshire Street
London W1N 1RJ
Tel: 020 7935 2163
Will forward list of practitioners on receipt of large A4 SAE, 60p stamp.
Open 1.30 pm-5 pm

British Infertility Counselling Association (BICA)
69 Division Street
Sheffield S1 4GE
Tel: 01342 843880
Provides lists of fertility counsellors, hosts educational events and produces
quarterly *Journal of Fertility Counselling*
Web site: http://www.bica.net

British Menopause Society
36 West Street
Marlow
Buckinghamshire SL7 2NB
Tel: 01628 890 199
Professional society offering information and publishes *Journal of the
British Menopause Society*

British Psychology Society (BPS)
St Andrews House
48 Princess Road East
Leicester LE1 7DR
Tel: 0116 254 9568
Fax: 0116 247 0787
e-mail: mail@bps.org.uk
Web site: http://www.bps.org.uk
Lists of chartered, clinical and counselling psychologists available

Child
Charter House
43 St Leonards Road
Bexhill on Sea
East Sussex TN40 1JA
Tel: 01424 732361
Fax:01424 731858
e-mail: office@email2.child.org.uk
Web site: http://www.child.org.uk
National self-help network for those trying for a family; carries books on the subject

Child Link
10 Lion Yard
Tremadoc Road
London SW4 7NQ
Tel: 020 7498 1933
Fax: 020 7498 1791
Voluntary adoption agency

COTS
Loandhu Cottage
Gruids
Lairg
Sutherland
Scotland IV27 4EF
Tel: 01549 402401
Agency specializing in surrogacy arrangements; provides information and counselling

DI Network
PO Box 265
Sheffield S3 7YX
Group of parents who are undergoing donor insemination treatment and/or whose children were born from donated gametes. Offers practical and emotional support to parents about telling their children about their origins, and enables parents and children to meet others in the same position

Early Menopause Clinic
John Radcliffe Hospital
Oxford OX3 9DU
Includes infertility specialists and endocrinologists as well as menopause specialists. Needs referral from GP

FORESIGHT, Association for the Promotion of Pre-Conceptual Care
28 The Paddock
Godalming
Surrey GU7 1XD
Tel: 01483 427839
Fax: 01483 427668
Offers a video, booklets and leaflets on non-technological approaches to fertility issues

Faculty of Homeopathy
Homeopathic Trust
15 Clerkenwell Close
London EC1R 0AA
Tel: 020 7566 7800
Fax: 020 7566 7815
Will provide information (including two papers on menopause on request) and a list of registered, medically-trained homeopaths plus well known homeopathic suppliers and manufacturers if sent a large SAE

Human Fertilisation & Embryology Authority (HFEA)
Paxton House
30 Artillery Lane
London E1 7LS
Tel: 020 7377-5077
Fax: 020 7377-1871
Statutory body responsible for licensing fertility clinics in the UK. Produces information leaflets, e.g. on egg donation, and can provide a list of clinics offering egg donation

Hysterectomy Association
Aynsley House
Chester Gardens
Church Gresley
Swadlincote
Derbyshire DE11 9PU
Web site: http://www.hysterectomy-association.org.uk/index.htm

The Institute of Psychosexual Medicine
11 Chandos Street
Cavendish Square
London W1M 9DE
Tel: 020 7580 0631

ISSUE, The National Fertility Association
509 Aldridge Rd
Great Bart
Birmingham B44 8NA
Tel: 01922 72288
National fertility support organisation that gives advice and information to members about infertility treatments and services. Has regional support groups and a regular newsletter

Lupus UK
1 Eastern Road
Romford
Essex RM1 3NH
Tel: 01708 731 251
A self-help organization for people with lupus with support groups and contacts throughout the UK

Multiple Birth Foundation
Queen Charlotte & Chelsea Hospital
Goldhawk Road
London W6 OXG
Tel: 020 8748 4666
Offers free counselling service to parents and provide information and literature on
issues affecting multiples

National Endometriosis Society
Suite 50
Westminster Palace Gardens
1-7 Artillery Row
London SW1P 1RL
Helpline: 020 7222 2776
Offers information and support to women with endometriosis, a condition that can
disrupt the menstrual cycle

National Institute of Medical Herbalists
56 Longbrook Street
Exeter
Devon EX4 6AH
Tel: 01392 426022
Will send list of members and publications, including bibliography on receipt of
Stamped self-addressed envelope

**National Organisation for the Counselling of Adoptees and their Parents
(NORCAP)**
3 New High Street
Headington
Oxford OX3 7AJ
Tel: 01865 750554
Support group to help adults handle their feelings about the effect of adoption on their
lives. Publishes quarterly magazine. Contact leaders are available throughout the coun-
try and may arrange meetings for local members

National Osteoporosis Society
PO Box 10
Radstock
Bath BA3 3YB
Tel: 01761 471771
Fax: 01761 471104
Helpline: 01761 472721
Web site: http://www.pslgroup.com/osteoporosis.htm
Registered charity offering independent information on osteoporosis, menopause,
HRT, exercises and a publications list

Ovacome (Ovarian Cancer Support Network)
St Bartholomew's Hospital
West Smithfield
London EC1A 7BE
Tel: 0207 1781 861
Web site: http://www.dspace.dial.pipex.com/ovacome

Overseas Adoption Helpline
PO Box 13899
London N6 4WB
Tel: 0990 168 742 (Mon–Fri 9 am–1 pm/2 pm–5 pm)
Fax: 020 8348 1522
Provides written information leaflets (cost from £3–£20) on different countries and general procedures as well as telephone advice

Overseas Adoption Support and Information Service (OASIS)
c/o Coral Williams
Dan-y-graig Cottage
Balaclava Road
Glais
Swansea SA7 9HJ
Tel: 01792 844329

Parent to Parent Information on Adoption Services (PPIAS)
Lower Bodington
Daventry
Northamptonshire NN11 6YB
Tel: 01327 260295
Fax: 01327 263565
Provides information, contacts and support for prospective parents and professionals

Pituitary Foundation
PO Box 1944
Bristol BS99 2UB
e-mail: helpline@pitpat.demon.co.uk

Post Adoption Centre
8 Torriano Mews
Torriano Avenue
London NW5 2RZ
Tel: 020 7284 0555
Fax: 020 7482 2367
Confidential counselling service for anyone involved in adoption, pre and post adoption

Pre-Adoption Counselling & Consultancy Service
28 Cranley Gardens
London N10 3AP
Tel: 020 8444 8084

Turner Syndrome Society
1/8 Irving Court
Hardgate
Clydebank G81 6BA
Tel: 01389 380385
Web site: http://www.tss.org.uk

UK Turner Syndrome Society
c/o Child Growth Foundation
2 Mayfield Avenue
London W4 1PW
Provides information, advice and support for parents of Turner Syndrome girls and adult women with the syndrome and publishes a newsletter. Send a self-addressed stamped envelope for information

Women's Health Concern
93–99 Upper Richmond Road
London SW15 2TG
Tel: 020 8780 3007
Provides largely written information on menopause and HRT, plus some counselling by nurses in London, Newcastle-upon-Tyne, Surbiton and Peterborough

Women's Health Information Centre
52 Featherstone Street
London EC1Y 8RT
Tel: 020 7251 6580
e-mail: womenshealth@pop3.poptel.org.uk
Provides information and newsletter on women's health. Newsletter 34, September 1997, is on premature menopause

USA

Adoptive Families of America
333 Hwy 100 North
Minneapolis
MN 5542
Tel: (001) 612 537 0316
Largest organization for adoptive parents in the world; provides referrals to local parent groups

American Fertility Society (AFS)
1209 Montgomery Highway
Birmingham
AL 35216-2809
Tel: (001) 315 724 4348
International association of professionals with special interest in fertility

American Society for Reproductive Medicine
Suite 203
408 12th Street SW
Washington DC 20024-2125
Tel: (001) 212 863 2439
Fax: (001) 212 484 4039
Web site: http://www.asrm.com
Organisation for professionals interested in family planning and reproductive health, providing pamphlets on range of topics

The Childfree Network
1800-777 Sunset Boulevard
Citrus Heights
CA 95610
Tel: (001) 916 773 7178
Quarterly newsletter with articles on the beneficial and practical facets of life without children

Endometriosis Association (USA)
8585 N 76th Place
Milwaukee
WI 53223
Web site: http://www.endometriosisassoc.org/

National Council for Adoption
1930 17th St NW
Washington DC 20009
Tel: (001) 202 328 1200
Fax: (001) 202 322 0935
e-mail: ncfadc@ibm.net
Web site: http://www.ncfa-usa.org
Adoption advocacy organization with referrals to member agencies for traditional, confidential adoptions

National Osteoporosis Foundation (USA)
Suite 500
1150 17th St North West
Washington DC 20036-4603

North American Council on Adoptable Children (NACAC)
106-970 Raymond Avenue
St Paul
MN 5514-1149
Tel: (001) 612 644 3036
Advocates for special needs adoption. Publishes newsletter 'Adoptalk', provides information and list of adoption and related resources including web sites

Organization of Parents Through Surrogacy (OPTS)
National Headquarters
PO Box 611
Gurnee
IL 60031
Tel: (001) 847 782 0224
Fax: (001) 847 782 0240
Web site: http://ww.opts.com
National non-profit organization run by volunteers providing mutual support, network-
ing and information, including directory of agencies, attorneys, physicians and psycho-
logical professionals plus newsletter

Parents of Only Children
4719 Reed Road
Suite 121
Columbus
OH 43220
Tel: (001) 614- 442 0873
Organisation promoting communication among only children, their parents, spouses
and friends, plus professionals dedicated to influencing societal attitudes towards only
children

POF Support Group
PO Box 23643
Alexandria
VA 22304
e-mail: pof2@aol.com
Web site: http://www.POFSupport.org

Resolve Inc
1310 Broadway
Sommerville
MA 02144-1731
Tel: (001) 617 623- 1156 (office)
Fax: (001) 617 623 0252
Helpline (001) 617 623 0744
Web site: http://www.resolve.org
Provides education, support and advocacy services with chapters nationwide

Turner's Syndrome Society of the US
Suite 327
1313 South East 5th Street
Minneapolis
MN 55414
Web site: http://www.turner-syndrome-us.org/

Canada

Turner's Syndrome Society of Canada
814 Glencairn Avenue
Toronto
Ontario M6B 2A3

Web sites

Overview of women's health
http://cpmcnet.columbia.edu/dept/rosenthal

Menopause
http://www.pslgroup.com/menopause.htm
http://www.howdyneighbor.com/menopaus/
http://www.oxford.net/~tishy/elists.html
http://www.daisychain.org/
http://www.members.aol.com/MenoChat/#Anchor-47857

Surgical menopause
http://www.findins.net/sans-uteri.html
http://www.endometriosis.org
http://members.tripod.com/fiona_51

UK Adoption web site
http://www.rainbowkids.com

Index